Rapid Internal Medicine Board Review and Recertification Guide

OWN THE BOARDS

Rapid Internal Medicine Board Review and Recertification Guide

Cyrus Peikari, MD

Department of Internal Medicine
Presbyterian Hospital
Dallas, TX

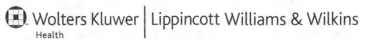

Wolters Kluwer | Lippincott Williams & Wilkins
Health

Philadelphia • Baltimore • New York • London
Buenos Aires • Hong Kong • Sydney • Tokyo

Acquisitions Editor: Sonya Seigafuse
Managing Editor: Nancy Winter
Marketing Manager: Kimberly Schonberger
Production Editor: Bridgett Dougherty
Manufacturing Manager: Kathleen Brown
Design Coordinator: Stephen Druding
Compositor: ITC
Printer: R R Donnelley Crawfordsville

Library of Congress Cataloging-in-Publication Data

Peikari, Cyrus.
Own the boards : rapid internal medicine board review and recertification
guide / Cyrus Peikari.
p. ; cm.
Includes index.
ISBN-13: 978-0-7817-7215-0
ISBN-10: 0-7817-7215-X
1. Internal medicine—Examinations, questions, etc.   2. American Board of
Internal Medicine—Examinations—Study guides.   I. Title.   II. Title: Rapid
internal medicine board review and recertification guide.
[DNLM: 1. Internal Medicine—Outlines.   WB 18.2 P377o 2008]
RC58.P42 2008
616.0076–dc22

                                                            2007008560

Dr. Cyrus Peikari is humbled before Bahá'u'lláh ("Glory of God"), the prophet-founder of the Baha'i Faith. He also thanks his students, teachers, and fellow seekers of knowledge. Dr. Peikari is also grateful to his family for their constant support and encouragement.

CONTENTS

PREFACE

This book is a high-yield, rapid review for the ABIM Internal Medicine Board and Recertification Exam. The content is derived primarily from interviewing hundreds of physicians immediately after sitting for their Board exams. Without revealing specific questions or exam material, these physicians gave clues as to which topics seem to be emphasized time and again on the Boards.

The material in this book is derived from the live "Own the Boards" Internal Medicine Review Course presented by Dr. Peikari each year in Dallas, TX (www.owntheboards.com). This material has been classroom tested by hundreds of physicians who have attended the live course over the last few years. By interviewing these physicians after their exams, the review has been optimized and fine-tuned.

There is no fluff or filler in this book. This is Board review in its most distilled form. If a topic is covered here, then something similar was probably asked on a recent Board exam. On the other hand, that means that this book is not comprehensive. There will be material on your exam that is not covered in this rapid-fire guide. For this reason, in the text we recommend additional study resources to round out your review.

In order to save time, this book assumes that you know the basics of internal medicine and primary care. We don't re-hash the medical treatment of routine diabetes, hypertension, or hyperlipidema. Instead, we focus on more esoteric material that you might not use on a daily basis. You'll learn more about Addison disease, Wegener granulomatosis, and Still disease, to name a few examples.

The goal of this book is to boost your scores enough to pass the exam with ease. Sadly, most physicians who fail the exam do so by only 5 or 10 questions. The ABIM grades your exam on an arbitrary, pre-determined passing score, rather than correcting it with a curve. And their passing margins are very narrow. In fact, most physicians who do not pass the exam are heartbroken to find that just a handful of key questions would have saved them. Fortunately, this book should push you far beyond merely passing.

But is it really useful to get feedback from physicians who have just taken the exam? Yes! In fact, most major review courses do this to refine their material. For example, several major, university-based courses have been using this method for years. However, not everyone can afford to pay a week's tuition, not to mention airfare, hotel, and lost income from work. The total expenses to attend a one-week, review course easily can exceed $5,000.

Even the American College of Physicians (ACP) uses physician feedback to refine their material. On their website, the ACP advertises that their review gives an "advantage" in part because they "surveyed more than 200 associate members of the ACP shortly after they completed the American Board of Internal Medicine (ABIM) certifying examination." However, the ACP materials can be expensive, costing up to several hundred dollars.

These weeklong, fly-in review courses, and media packages such as the ACP's, are unquestionably useful. However, not everyone can afford to spend that much time and money; except, perhaps, for some of the wealthier sub-specialists. But for the general internist who is in the trenches, it's too costly. Between managing a busy practice, and paying society dues, malpractice insurance, and other overhead, it's just not in the budget. So the humble internist is at a disadvantage. That is, until now.

This book levels the playing field by bringing the same information into the hands of the practicing internist. Now you can get a thorough review while still keeping up with the demands of your busy practice. The information here is presented in bite-sized chunks. This design allows you to review during lunch, after work, or even between patients at the office.

There are a few unique features to this book. For example, some review books try to be "all things to all students." They may cram in as many tables, facts, and mnemonics as they can. But instead of helping, this data overload is just confusing—especially since the Boards now focus on clinical vignettes. It's hard enough keeping ten thousand medical facts in your brain, right? Now imagine sorting through them every 90 seconds as you race through questions on the exam! For this reason, long and tricky mnemonics can just be confusing. Some of us just want the bare facts, with a minimum of bells and whistles.

Another advantage of this book is its emphasis on solving formula problems. After completing this book, you will know how to solve certain formula questions with almost perfect accuracy. For example, nearly every Board exam includes questions on Bayes theorem, as well as questions on triple acid-base disorders. Many physicians learn this material briefly in medical school and residency, but then quickly forget it because they never again need it in practice. And many review books tuck this information in at the end, almost as an afterthought, so that you never really learn it. In contrast, this book clearly and plainly will show you how to solve these problems with ease. We even include "homework" assignments to make sure you really master the material. After reading this book you should never miss one of these questions again. It's like adding free bonus points to your exam score. As one physician recently wrote:

I just wanted to let you know I passed the ABIM recertification exam by ten questions. Thanks to your review, I know I got all the acid base questions and probability questions right. That alone was almost enough to put me over the top. Thanks!

The website provides images (such as hematology and dermatology slides) similar to those that may appear on your Board exam. Your exam is computer based, so you had better get used to looking at digital images, rather than print.

This book is a condensed, highly targeted review that you can finish quickly. It will help any physician who is studying for the ABIM Internal Medicine Board Exam for either initial certification or recertification. It will also help internal medicine residents who are preparing to take their in-service exams. Some have even found it useful in preparing for the internal medicine portions of the Step III exams. If you want to ratchet your Board score several points upward, as quickly as possible, then this book is for you.

ACKNOWLEDGMENTS

The author would like to thank the following technical reviewers who helped to improve the text.

Those who probably deserve the most credit, but who for privacy reasons are not listed here, are the hundreds of physicians who have attended the live "Own the Boards" review course. Their kind feedback, both during the course and then immediately after taking the ABIM exam, is what adds the most value to this book.

P. Terrence Moore, M.D.
Neurology and Sleep Medicine
Department of Medicine
Presbyterian Hospital
Allen, TX

Sumit Kumar, M.D.
Department of Nephrology
Presbyterian Hospital
Dallas, TX

Kousik Krishnan, M.D., FACC
Assistant Professor of Medicine
Director, Arrhythmia Device Clinic
Associate Director, Electrophysiology Laboratory
Rush University Medical Center
Chicago, Illinois

Julia Liaci, M.D., MPH
Department of Obstetrics and Gynecology
Presbyterian Hospital
Dallas, TX

Rajeev Jain, M.D.
Department of Gastroenterology
Presbyterian Hospital
Dallas, TX

Sandeep Gupta, M.D.
Department of Allergy and Immunology
Presbyterian Hospital
Dallas, TX

Michael A. Tolle, M.D.
Baylor International Pediatric AIDS Initiative
Texas Children's Hospital
Houston, TX
Lesotho Children's Clinic,
Maseru, Lesotho

Gebre Tseggay, M.D.
Department of Infectious Disease
Presbyterian Hospital
Dallas, TX

Julye Carew, M.D.
Pulmonary and Critical Care Medicine
Presbyterian Hospital
Dallas, TX

Kiran Kancharla, M.D.
Department of Hematology and Oncology
Presbyterian Hospital
Dallas, TX

CHAPTER 1

Study Tips and Test Tricks

You have a 10%–15% chance of failing the Boards on your first attempt. At least, that is the typical failure rate published by the American Board of Internal Medicine (ABIM) in any given year. However, with the information in this book, you can help stack the odds in your favor.

The ABIM currently uses a fixed, pre-determined cutoff score to determine passing. This number is arbitrarily chosen, and it is based on what they consider will demonstrate a "competent" internist. In contrast, other nationwide, standardized tests (such as the college-entrance S.A.T. exam) have moved to a system of grading on a curve. In other words, the S.A.T. statistically balances the scores to make sure the relative difficulty is consistent from year to year.

Perhaps the ABIM should consider grading on a curve. That might help to pick out the real outliers—the physicians who fail the test by a large margin and who clearly should not be practicing. But for right now, the Board's arbitrary cutoff fails 10%–15% or more physicians each time. Many of those who fail may, in reality, be more experienced and qualified practitioners than some who pass; these physicians might fail only because they are not expert test takers.

The Board exam also does not take into account different practice styles. For example, in your practice you can do an Internet search on a rare disease, and within two minutes you will know a great deal about its diagnosis, treatment, and differential. In this respect, the Board exam misses the reality of modern practice—and ignores the power that the Internet brings to physicians.

Perhaps things will change in the future. For now, however, you are stuck with the old, sometimes brutal, grading method. But you should not be discouraged. Reviewing for the Boards can be exhilarating and even pleasurable. During the course of your review, you will gain more confidence than you have ever had. The review will feed your hungry intellect. And you may even stumble across the diagnoses to some rare and difficult patient cases that have eluded you until now.

How to use this book

Ideally, you will have at least three to four weeks to master this book. However, in a pinch it can be finished in just one week—if you are willing to clear extra hours each day in your schedule.

Chapter 2 (Questions You Should Never Miss) is the only chapter where you really have to turn on your brain. For this chapter you should find a couple of hours in a quiet library or in your office after everyone has gone home. You cannot have any distractions whatsoever, including children, pets, or even phone or Internet access. This is the chapter where you will have to do some problem solving, just like you did back in high-school algebra. It is probably the strongest chapter of this book, and you will be selling yourself short if you don't take it seriously.

The rest of the book can be studied "on the fly": at lunch, in the evenings at home, or even between patients during a slow office day. No learning is required for this material—just rote memorization. Think back to medical school when you had to "flash burn" hundreds of pages of lecture notes into your brain every week. Unlike medical school, however, you can now go at your own pace and with less pressure. You might even enjoy it.

Remember that the ABIM has its own idea of what is "rare" and what is "common." For example, Wegener granulomatosis might show up four times on your exam. However, outside of residency, you might not see a Wegener case more than four times in your entire career! This book will reflect the ABIM's peculiarities. We will emphasize rare points about common diseases, and common points about some rare diseases.

Most chapters in this book are simply rapid-fire bullet points. These bullets contain the highlights of questions that were asked on recent Board exams. The best way to read the book is with a pen in hand. The first time you read through the book, go slowly. On this first pass, put a check mark in front of any bullet that is new to you.

The second time you read through the book, switch to a red pen. This time, read only the bullets that already have a check mark in front of them. However, if there was a point that you didn't remember clearly from the first time through, then add a second check mark in front of it;—this time in red.

On the third and final pass, simply glance through the red-checked bullets. Make sure you have them memorized. If you have time, you might even go through the book for a fourth and a fifth time. However, by that point you should be able to breeze through the entire book in just a couple of well-focused hours. These final passes may seem very quick and perfunctory, but they help to "flash" the information into your short- and medium-term memory.

Study plan

Alone, this book is not enough to pass the boards safely. You need to "cross train" with different review books. It's like a marathon runner who does only one kind of training run: It is difficult to win a marathon with such poor preparation. A good runner, in contrast, will mix up the training routine with hills, fast and slow runs, and even cross training with weights.

A good example of a supplemental guide is the *Cleveland Clinic Intensive Review of Internal Medicine*. Be warned: it's huge! Weighing in at nearly 1,000 pages, this guide works best if you have at least three to six months of study time, but if time is short, simply pick and choose the parts that you read. Use it to review and strengthen your weakest sections. Another good review is the *Medical Knowledge Self-Assessment Program® (MKSAP)* materials; however, most physicians who buy it report that they simply don't have time to go into that much depth.

Finally, it is important to do practice test questions. *Harrison's Principles of Internal Medicine* has a spin-off book offering more than 1,000 sample questions. The *Cleveland Clinic* review, mentioned above, has many good questions as well. Always, always, always time yourself when taking practice questions. If you do not train under the clock, then you are likely to run out of time during the real exam.

Just like a marathon runner who rarely runs a full marathon in training, you should never take an entire six hour practice test at one sitting. Thirty or sixty questions at a time are enough. Trying to take an entire day's worth of practice tests could lead to "overtraining." This is a disastrous form of burnout. If you can relax and have fun with your studying, then you will do better on exam day.

Repeating the test

If you have failed the ABIM exam once before, and you are trying to retake it, then the single most important thing you can do is to study with a partner. This is crucial. You *must* study with someone else. It is the only way to ensure that you are absorbing the material. The best way might be to make a schedule and then review a chapter or two each night by yourself; the next day you would then take turns quizzing each other on that material. In just three or four weeks, you will probably change a near-failing score to an easily passing one. If you really want to pass your second attempt, you cannot afford to skip this advice.

Pre-game preparation

A professional runner does not run the day before a marathon. Likewise, you should not try to study anything on the day before the exam. After absorbing thousands of facts, your brain needs this "air gap" in order to consolidate what you recently memorized with what you had previously learned.

It is also a good idea to exercise the day before the exam, if you are able. A number of physicians are so worried about the exam that they stay up all night and don't sleep properly before the test. As a result, they fail horribly. Exercise can exhaust your body so that you will sleep soundly before the exam. Exercise will also burn off a large part of your stress.

On the day of the exam, you should bring your own food (and your own caffeine, if needed). Don't think that you will have time to run out to a fast food chain, because there might not be any nearby. And it will be more energizing if you eat light food that you have prepared yourself. You should plan to eat and drink a little bit between every section of the exam.

You should also stretch and walk during the breaks. Also, during the breaks, do not discuss the test questions with anyone. Not only will this get your test invalidated, but it can also raise your anxiety level. There are still a few gunners out there who mistakenly believe that trying to "psyche out" the other test takers will somehow improve their score on a national exam. Tell yourself that this is *your* day—you are alone, and no one else exists.

Taking the test When taking the exam, you should work straight through. Don't skip questions. Try to answer short questions in 60 seconds and longer ones in 90 seconds. Of course, this is an ideal, because some questions will take more than two minutes. The clinical vignettes are getting longer each year. So you need to store extra time on the easy questions when you can.

If there is a question about which you are not 100% sure, mark it and come back to it at the end of the section. Computer-based testing makes this easy, and you will automatically be taken back to these marked questions once you have finished. Hopefully, you have left enough time for a quick review. But don't talk yourself out of a correct answer. Your first choice is likely to be the correct choice; trust your intuition, unless you have a really good reason for changing the answer.

Some test takers prefer to read the "lead line" before reading the question. The lead line is the final line in the question, right before the choices are presented. You may choose to do this only occasionally. For example, if you are getting drowsy towards the end of the exam, starting with the lead line can help wake you up.

Try to answer the question in your head before reading any of the choices. And make sure to read all the possible answers before making a choice. If you just pick the first choice that sounds good, chances are you have missed a better answer just below it. Also, look for the "giveaway" questions. For example, seeing the word "anosmia" in a question should make you think of Kallmann syndrome; "lancinating" pain is unique to trigeminal neuralgia; and the words "Bakersfield, California" guarantee coccidiomycosis.

Mastering computer-based testing

You will take your exam on a computer. This can sound scary, but it actually provides a number of advantages. For example, you can automatically mark the questions about which you are unsure; the computer will automatically take you back to these for easy review at the end of each section.

You should also remember that using a typical computer monitor is like staring into a 60-watt light bulb. Imagine staring into a light bulb for six straight hours. You are bound to get blurred vision and a headache. In fact, some physicians get migraines during the exam, occasionally severe enough that they have to quit. The solution to this is to master the computer when you first sit down. The monitor will have brightness and contrast adjustment controls. The test center will allow you to adjust the brightness until it is comfortable for you. In fact, you should turn both the brightness and contrast settings down as far as they will go, or as dim as you can get while still being able to read the material. Note that you will want to turn the brightness back up, for a few moments, whenever you get to a question with an image.

Reading digital images

While we are on the subject of images, there is a key point to remember: computer-based images look very different from printed images. For example, a color atlas of dermatology may be able to print an image with millions of subtle color variations. In contrast, the images on your computer-based test have been digitally compressed, and they are stripped of much of their color. Furthermore, most test centers use less expensive, low-end graphics cards and monitors. This further degrades the computer image when compared to a print image. Your eye can sense the difference.

For this reason, we have not printed color plates in this book. Instead, we have compiled an online bank of digital images. This study tool will help to reinforce the images that you may be likely to see on your Board exam. By reviewing them in digital form, your eye will become trained in reading computer-based images.

In addition, you can search for images on your own. Most Internet search engines have "image searches." Simply enter the name of the disease or condition, and you will instantly find hundreds of images that match your search. In this way, you can see a wide variety of examples of the same condition. This variety will help to burn the image into your mind, and it can give you a significant advantage on the exam.

The obligatory disclaimer

Be warned: you should not try to use the material in this book for diagnosing and treating real patients. We suggest you consult a medical textbook for that. Similar to the Board exam itself, this book does not reflect actual practice. This is a compressed, highly targeted review. The goal is to help you score some easy points that otherwise you might have missed. To this end, we have deliberately left off background, workup, treatment, etc. on many diseases. If a fact wasn't on a recent Board exam, then you probably won't find it in here.

While every effort was made to ensure the accuracy of this book, there will always be errors. Errata, as well as the latest updates, will be posted online at www.owntheboards.com. While you're at the website, please take the time to email the author. Your helpful comments can be published online for the benefit of other test takers. Remember, feedback from you (the reader) is what keeps this material fresh and vital.

Now relax, have fun, and enjoy the book!

CHAPTER 2

Questions You Should Never Miss

Nearly every Board exam has certain "formula" problems that appear again and again. Examples are triple acid-base disorders, Bayes theorem problems, and Number Needed to Treat (NNT) calculations. The good news is that these problems are easy points if you know how to solve them. The bad news is that very few of us remember what we learned about them in medical school, and there seem to be very few (if any) resources that explain them really well.

By the end of this chapter, you should be able to solve all of these problem types with nearly 100% accuracy. But you're going to have to do a bit of work. Think back to high-school algebra or college calculus. Remember that the best way to learn math problems is to struggle in trying to solve them on your own—before looking at the answers. If you skip the painful part and just read the solutions instead, then you will never really learn it. You need a math-homework mindset in order to work through this chapter. In fact, at the end of the chapter are some extra "homework" problems for you to solve at a later date. This will help you master the material.

Remember, for many people a mere handful of questions will determine whether they pass the Boards. Since these formula questions are almost sure to be on your exam, it is worth taking a few hours to learn them. It could be that extra push over the top that you need. In contrast, if you skip this material or blow it off, it could come back to haunt you. There is nothing more disappointing that having to repeat the exam. So let's add these weapons to your arsenal.

Bayes theorem

Bayes theorem is a long, mathematical formula that most of us remember from medical school or from college statistics classes. None of us remember the exact formula, and few of us even remember how to construct the 2 × 2 tables. Yet we all use Bayes in our daily practice, usually subconsciously.

For example, when you see a patient with chest pain, you need to risk-stratify them by ordering some sort of cardiac evaluation. For a young, healthy patient with atypical chest pain, you might order a simple treadmill ECG stress test. That is because you know that the prevalence of coronary artery disease is low in this population. Thus, your pre-test probability is low. So you just need a safe, simple screening test with adequate sensitivity. You are trying to rule them "out," rather than ruling them "in" for cardiac disease.

In contrast, an elderly patient with multiple risk factors (diabetes, hypertension, and smoking, for example), who presents with classic angina, needs a more specific test. In this case, you are not trying to rule them out, since from their history you are almost certain that they have critical coronary blockages. In fact, if you did a simple treadmill ECG stress test, and it came out normal (e.g., a false negative), then you would have wasted the patient's time and money. In this case, you would go straight for the coronary angiogram to get a definitive diagnosis.

Bayes theorem simply places the above subconscious, mental calculation into a more formal, mathematical equation. It describes the relationship between prevalence and the predictive value. *Bayes theorem states that the predictive value of a given diagnostic test is related to its pre-test prevalence in the population.*

For the purposes of the Board, you will have to memorize the following simplified formulas. You will also have to remember how to draw a 2 × 2 table (Table 1) from scratch. To make sure you have learned this material, after finishing this chapter you should put it aside; then, pull out these problems again in a couple of days, and try to solve them using a blank piece of paper. It is also worth writing out these formulas during the week, whenever you get a free moment. That is because on the test you will have to write it all out again, very quickly, from memory.

NOTE: On the ABIM exam, even though it is now computer-based, you will be provided with a small, erasable whiteboard. This will allow you to write out formulas and to perform calculations.

Table 1	The Bayes theorem 2 × 2 table that must be memorized.	
	Condition Present	Condition Absent
Test Positive	True Positive A	False Positive B
Test Negative	False Negative C	True Negative D
	Total # with condition	Total # without condition

Bayes formulas

The following formulas must be committed to memory. However, using the 2 × 2 table you have already memorized in Table 1, you can use a graphical trick to memorize them.

FORMULA 2-1: SENSITIVITY
- Sensitivity = A / (A + C)

FORMULA 2-2: SPECIFICITY
- Specificity = D / (B + D)

FORMULA 2-3: PREVALENCE
- Prevalence = (A + C) / (A + B + C + D)

The following questions also show up frequently, so you should learn them as well:

FORMULA 2-4: POSITIVE PREDICTIVE VALUE
- Positive Predictive Value = A / (A + B)

FORMULA 2-5: NEGATIVE PREDICTIVE VALUE
- Negative Predictive Value = D / (C + D)

NOTE: Please take a moment to pull out a blank piece of paper and a pencil right now. Then close this book, and try to write out the above 2 × 2 table, and all the above formulas, completely from memory. Do not give up and open the book until you have tried for at least two full minutes.

Example 2-1: Bayes analysis

In the following example you will use what you have memorized to solve a Bayes theorem problem.

Table 2	Sample 2 × 2 table used in Example 2-1.	
HIV Test Results	Antibody Present	Antibody Absent
Positive	98	3
Negative	2	297

Example 2-1: Using the 2 × 2 table in Table 2, calculate the Sensitivity, Specificity, and Prevalence.

After you have copied Example 2-1 to a blank piece of paper, close this book and try to solve it on your own. Your first step will be to write out the formulas from memory. Do not give up or open this book to look at the solution until at least five minutes have passed. Even if you can't remember anything, simply struggle with the blank piece of paper and a pencil as best you can.

Example 2-1 solution
Did you get it? Don't worry if you didn't. Most people get stuck at this early point. Using Formulas 2-1, 2-2, and 2-3, we can add in the appropriate values from the 2 × 2 table in Table 2.

That gives us the following results:

$$\text{Sensitivity} = A / (A + C)$$
$$= 98 / (98 + 2) = .98$$
$$\text{Specificity} = D / (B + D)$$
$$= 297 / (297 + 3) = .99$$
$$\text{Prevalence} = (A + C) / (A + B + C + D)$$
$$= (98 + 2) / (98 + 3 + 2 + 297)$$
$$= (100) / (400)$$
$$= .25$$

We thus have a sensitivity of 98%, a specificity of 99%, and a prevalence of 25%.

Example 2-2: Working backwards

Just when you were getting comfortable, we are going to make it harder. Board questions often ask you to work the above problem in reverse, which is more difficult.

Example 2-2: Your test has a sensitivity of 98% and specificity of 99%. If the prevalence of HIV in your target population is 25%, then what percent of patients testing positive will actually have the disease?

Again, take out a fresh, blank piece of paper and a pencil. You will need to draw your own 2 × 2 table from memory, in addition to writing out the formulas from memory. You may have no idea how to answer this type of question. Nevertheless, try to work something out on your own. Do not open this book until you have struggled on your own for at least five minutes.

Example 2-2 solution
Did you get the answer? No? Well, neither did anyone else who has reached this point in the chapter. There is a certain trick to it.

First, we will draw out our 2 × 2 table from memory as shown in Table 3. As you can see in Table 3, we have arbitrarily put in a total number of patients as 400. How did we come up with this number? We just picked it randomly. It's arbitrary. The exact value doesn't matter. Some people who solve the problem pick 1,000, some pick 100, some pick 200, etc.

This is the part that confuses most people. It takes a leap of faith to pick an arbitrary number for a total. But after you have done it a few times, it will seem easy and natural to you. And you will find yourself picking numbers that are easiest for you to solve.

Now that we have picked 400 as our arbitrary total, we can "work backwards." If we know that our total is 400, and that our prevalence is 25% (or 0.25), we can calculate the total number with the condition as (0.25) × 400 = 100. You can look back at Table 1 to remember how this all fits together. Since there is a total of 400, and 100 of them are in the left-sided column, it means that 400 − 100 = 300 are left over. Thus, we put the remaining 300 in the middle column. Looking back at Table 1, these 300 are the total number of those who do not have the disease.

In Table 4, we continue working backwards and start to fill in the remaining blanks of our 2 × 2 table.

We know that our sensitivity is 98%. And we know from Table 1 and from Formula 2-1 how sensitivity is derived from the 2 × 2 table. Take

Table 3	Picking an arbitrary total and working backwards.		
HIV Test Results	Antibody Present	Antibody Absent	Total
Positive			
Negative			
Total	100	300	400

Table 4	Continuing to work backwards.		
HIV Test Results	Antibody Present	Antibody Absent	Total
Positive	98	3	101
Negative	2	297	299
Total	100	300	400

a moment to look at Table 1. And remember that Formula 2-1 tells us that sensitivity = A / (A + C). So working backwards, we put 98 in the "A" box of the 2 × 2 table (recall from Table 1 that the "A" box is in the upper left corner). That leaves 100 − 98 = 2 left over to complete the total number with the condition. The 2 that are left over go into the "C" box of Table 1 as false negatives.

We are now almost finished filling in Table 4. Can you see how the "C" and "D" boxes were filled? We know from Formula 2-2 that the Specificity = D / (B+D). Thus, working backwards we fill in (0.98) × 300 = 297. This leaves 3 left over. You can now see how these fit into Table 4.

Now we have filled in the entire table by cleverly working backwards. But what is the answer to the question? Example 2-2 is asking us *"What percent of patients testing positive will actually have the disease?"* You will have to learn that phrase as code for *"What is the positive predictive value?"* Looking back at Formula 2-4, we can now calculate that:

$$\text{Positive Predictive Value} = A / (A + B)$$
$$= 98 / (101)$$
$$= 97\%$$

In our example, that means that 97% of patients testing positive will actually have the disease.

Example 2-3: Bayes again

Now that you are an expert, try to solve the following question on your own, without looking at the answer.

Example 2-3: You know that in your study population the prevalence of breast cancer is 10%. Your mammogram has a sensitivity of 75% and

Table 5	Your numbers will probably be different than these.		
Mammogram Results	Disease Present	Disease Absent	Total
Positive	75	90	165
Negative	25	810	835
Total	100	900	1,000

a specificity of 90%. What percent of patients with a normal mammogram will *not* have cancer?

Close your book and try to work this problem. Don't worry if it takes you ten minutes or longer. The important thing is that you wrestle with it until you get it right.

Example 2-3 solution
This problem is nearly identical to Example 2-2. For variety, for this example we arbitrarily picked the number 1,000 for the total in our population. You probably picked something different. But as long as you work backwards properly, then the results will be the same. Table 5 shows the 2 × 2 table after we have filled it out by working backwards, using the method of Example 2-2.

Once the table is filled, we can calculate the answer. Example 2-3 asks us "*What percent of patients with a normal mammogram will not have cancer?*" This is code for "*What is the negative predictive value?*"

From Formula 2-5 we know that Negative Predictive Value = D / (C + D). Thus,

$$\text{Negative Predictive Value} = D / (D + C)$$
$$= 810 / (810 + 25)$$
$$= 97\%$$

In our example, that means that 97% of patients with a normal mammogram will *not* have cancer.

Number needed to treat (NNT)

Number needed to treat questions are the easiest points you will ever score on a Board exam. So be sure to read them carefully and to do them correctly. In fact, most of us simply solve them in our heads. However, Formula 2-6 shows the formal equation so that you can be sure that your mental calculations are correct.

FORMULA 2-6
- NNT = 1 / (pre − post)

In Formula 2-6, "pre" refers to the percent incidence before the drug is used, and "post" is the percent incidence afterwards. Example 2-4 will illustrate this. Take a minute to try to work it in your head first before using the formula.

Example 2-4: A new drug decreases mortality from 65% to 45% when taken for three years. What is the number of patients who need to be treated for three years in order to save one life?

Example 2-4 solution
Using Formula 2-6, we know that

$$\begin{aligned}
\text{NNT} &= 1 / (\text{pre} - \text{post}) \\
&= 1 / (.65 - .45) \\
&= 1 / (.2) \\
&= 5
\end{aligned}$$

Thus, the number that need to be treated for three years is five patients. Note that the time period of "three years" has no bearing on solving the equation. This time period could be any number at all.

Solving acid-base problems

On the ABIM exam, if you try to solve an acid-base problem in your head, you will probably get it wrong (unless you happen to be either a pulmonologist or a nephrologist). That is because the Board exam usually asks complex, triple acid-base disorders. And they always make the multiple-choice options as tricky as possible. So don't try to "wing it."

Very few of us ever have to solve formal acid-base problems in real, daily practice. It's something we memorized in medical school and residency, but then quickly forgot. In fact, you are about to memorize it again, and you will probably forget it again after the exam is over. However, the goal of this section is to take the pain and mystery out of the problem solving. We will give you step-by-step instructions so that you never have to struggle or miss another acid-base problem on an exam. You will actually enjoy solving them. You may even start praying for them to show up on your test—because you will be one of the lucky few who gets them correct every time.

NOTE: When solving acid-base problems, always do a "reality check." Make sure the acid-base disorder matches the patient's clinical status.

For example, if you see a patient who is unresponsive and in septic shock, and you find no acid base disorder, then something is clearly wrong with your calculation! Similarly, look for easy clues. For example, persistent vomiting should lead to volume depletion and a metabolic alkalosis. Furthermore, sepsis should make you look for an anion-gap metabolic acidosis.

FORMULA 2-7: SIMPLIFIED ALGORITHM FOR SOLVING ACID-BASE DISORDERS
This formula actually has five steps, which are as follows:

1. Identify the primary acid-base disorder . . . is it acidotic or alkalotic?
2. Is the primary problem respiratory or metabolic? (Respiratory changes pCO_2, and metabolic changes HCO_3.)
3. Calculate the anion gap. (If increased, patient has a "gap" metabolic acidosis.)
4. Calculate the delta anion gap. (DAG) = AG measured − AG normal (12).
5. Add DAG to HCO_3
   a. If normal, no other metabolic problems.
   b. If <20, hyperchloremic, metabolic acidosis is also present.
   c. If >26, metabolic alkalosis is present.

NOTE: For the purpose of this formula, we always assume that a "normal" anion gap is 12. We also assume the normal pCO_2 to be 40, and the normal serum HCO_3 to be 24. Using these same reference numbers will ensure a correct result every time.

NOTE: The "delta" anion gap is merely a derived number. It is a placeholder to make sure we get our calculations correct. For the purpose of the Boards, it is simply necessary to know how to calculate it as shown in the examples below.

Example 2-5: Using the acid-base algorithm

Example 2-5: What is the acid-base status of a 25-year-old female who has pneumonia and the following lab values?

> ABG: pH 7.55/ $PaCO_2$ 29 / PaO_2 64
> Venous (mEq/L): Na^+ 144, K^+ 3.0, Cl^- 97, CO_2 20

Before reading the solution, take a few minutes now to try to work this out on your own. Copy the question and the lab values onto a blank piece of paper. For this first try, we are going to let you "cheat" and look at the steps in Formula 2-7 while solving it.

Example 2–5 solution
Did you get the correct solution? Don't worry; this was just the first try. Using Forumla 2-7, we will go through each of the steps:

1. Identify the primary acid-base disorder . . . is it acidotic or alkalotic?
   7.55 is *alkalotic.*
2. Is the primary problem respiratory or metabolic? (Respiratory changes pCO_2, and metabolic changes HCO_3.)
   The primary change is *respiratory.* (pCO_2 changes more than bicarb.)
3. Calculate the anion gap. (If increased, patient has a "gap" metabolic acidosis.)
   The anion gap (AG) = 144 − (97 + 20) = 27
   (So you also have a "gap" *metabolic acidosis.*)
4. Calculate the delta anion gap (DAG) = AG measured − AG normal (12).
   The DAG calculation might be new to some people.
   Here we calculate the DAG = 27 − 12 = 15.
5. Add DAG to HCO_3.
   a. If normal, no other metabolic problems.
   b. If <20, hyperchloremic, metabolic acidosis is also present.
   c. If >26, metabolic alkalosis is present.
   DAG + bicarb = 15 + 20 = 35.
   (Note that this is >26, so we also have a *metabolic alkalosis.*)

Now go through your calculations and circle all the acid-base conditions on your piece of paper (we have italicized them for you in this example). Now, collecting all our circled (italicized) findings from Steps 1 through 5, we see that our patient has a respiratory alkalosis, an anion-gap metabolic acidosis, and a metabolic acidosis. It's a triple acid-base disorder!

Example 2-6

Copy the following question and lab values to a blank piece of paper. Then close your book and try to solve it from scratch, without looking at your notes or at Formula 2-7. Don't give up and read the solution until you have tried at least five or ten minutes on your own.

Example 2-6: A 65-year-old vomiting, uremic patient has the following lab values:

> **ABG: pH 7.53 / PaCO$_2$ 47 / HCO$_3$ 38**
> **Venous (mEq/L): Na$^+$ 153, K$^+$ 5.7, Cl$^-$ 89, CO$_2$ 42**

Example 2-6 solution
Did you get it? Don't worry: at this point, most of us still have to open up the book and peek at the steps again. But you will have it memorized soon. By following the steps in Formula 2-7 we get the following:

1. Identify the primary acid-base disorder . . . is it acidotic or alkalotic?

   7.53 is *alkalotic.*

2. Is the primary problem respiratory or metabolic? (Respiratory changes pCO$_2$, and metabolic changes HCO$_3$.)

   The primary change is *metabolic.* (Bicarb changes more than pCO$_2$.)

3. Calculate the anion gap. (If increased, patient has a "gap" metabolic acidosis.)

   AG = 153 − (89 + 42) = 22
   (So you also have a "gap" *metabolic acidosis.*)

4. Calculate the delta anion gap (DAG) = AG measured − AG normal (12).

   DAG = 22 − 12 = 10.

5. Add DAG to HCO$_3$.
   a. If normal, no other metabolic problems.
   b. If <20, hyperchloremic, metabolic acidosis is also present.
   c. If >26, metabolic alkalosis is present.

   DAG + bicarb = 10 + 42 = 52.
   (Greater than 26 confirms *metabolic alkalosis* that we already know.)

   Thus, the acid-base disorder is metabolic alkalosis and "gap" metabolic acidosis.

Example 2-7

Hopefully, you have got the trick now. Let's try it one more time to be sure. Copy the following problem and labs onto a blank piece of paper, and try to solve it from scratch. This time, let's add some time pressure: see if you can do it in under two minutes.

Example 2-7: A 60-year-old man on mechanical ventilation for 72 hours after a drug overdose has the following lab values:

> ABG: pH 7.50 / $PaCO_2$ 24
> Venous (mEq/L): Na^+ 144, K^+ 3.8, Cl^- 102, CO_2 19

Example 2-7 solution
From Formula 2-7 we calculate the following:

1. Identify the primary acid-base disorder . . . is it acidotic or alkalotic?
   7.50 is *alkalotic.*

2. Is the primary problem respiratory or metabolic? (Respiratory changes pCO_2, and metabolic changes HCO_3.)
   The primary change is *respiratory.* (pCO_2 changes more than bicarb.)

3. Calculate the anion gap. (If increased, patient has a "gap" metabolic acidosis.)
   AG = 144 − (102 + 19) = 23.
   (So you also have a "gap" *metabolic acidosis.)*

4. Calculate the delta anion gap (DAG) = AG measured − AG normal (12).
   DAG = 23 − 12 = 11.

5. Add DAG to HCO_3.
   a. If normal, no other metabolic problems.
   b. If <20, hyperchloremic, metabolic acidosis is also present.
   c. If >26, metabolic alkalosis is present.
   DAG + bicarb = 11 + 19 = 30.
   (Greater than 26 means there is also a *metabolic alkalosis.)*

Thus, this patient has a triple acid-base disorder: respiratory alkalosis, "gap" metabolic acidosis, and metabolic alkalosis.

Congratulations: You are now an expert at solving mixed acid-base disorders!

P-value

You probably first learned about the P-value in a statistics class that you took in college. The P-value is used in hypotheses testing. It reflects the probability that an observed difference between the intervention and control groups is due to chance alone if the null hypothesis is true.

In practical terms, the P-value will show whether or not a study has statistical significance. For the purposes of the Board exam, you simply need to know the following: *If the P-value is less than 0.05, then the study is considered statistically significant.*

In addition, the lower the P-value, the greater the statistical significance. For example, a P-value of 0.01 is even more statistically significant than a P-value of 0.05.

Confidence interval

The confidence interval represents a range of uncertainty about an estimate of a treatment effect. It is calculated from differences in outcomes of the treatment and control groups, along with the sample size of a study.

A typical confidence interval is 95%. For example, a 95% confidence interval calculated from a particular study has a 95% probability of including the true value of a treatment effect. For the purposes of the Board exam, you simply need to know the following: *If the 95% confidence interval does not cross zero, then the study is considered statistically significant.*

For example, a study with a 95% confidence interval of 0.4 to 1.8 is considered significant. However, a 95% confidence interval of −0.9 to 0.6 is considered to be *not* significant (since the interval crosses zero).

Finishing touches

After mastering this chapter, you should come back to it every week or two and re-do the problems from scratch on blank pieces of paper. Then, a couple of days before the exam make one final pass through a few of these questions. It will give you the power and confidence to solve formula problems with near-perfect accuracy. Don't forget to try the extra "homework" problems that are included for you to practice.

Homework problems

To give you extra practice, we have included the following section on "homework problems." You should solve these on your own. The answers are listed in the Appendix; but please make sure not to look at any answers until you have solved each problem on your own.

Homework problem #1

A 54-year-old with uremia and vomiting presents with the following labs. What is the acid-base status?

ABG: pH 7.4 / $PaCO_2$ 40 / PaO_2 84
Venous (mEq/L): Na^+ 144, K^+ 3.0, Cl^- 99, CO_2 24

Homework problem #2

A 50-year-old diabetic female presents with lethargy, confusion, and the following labs. What is the acid-base status?

ABG: pH 7.20 / $PaCO_2$ 60
Venous (mEq/L): Na^+ 144, K^+ 3.1, Cl^- 99, CO_2 22

Homework problem #3

An 18-year-old diabetic male presents with obtundation and the following labs. What is the acid-base status?

ABG: pH 7.18 / $PaCO_2$ 30
Venous (mEq/L): Na^+ 142, K^+ 3.4, Cl^- 108, CO_2 10

Homework problem #4

A 44-year-old female presents with anorexia, vomiting, and tachypnea. What is the acid-base status?

ABG: pH 7.55 / $PaCO_2$ 18
Venous (mEq/L): Na^+ 143, K^+ 3.1, Cl^- 102, CO_2 16

Homework problem #5

A 17-year-old female presents with an unknown drug overdose. What is the acid-base status?

ABG: pH 7.49 / $PaCO_2$ 14
Venous (mEq/L): Na^+ 143, K^+ 3.1, Cl^- 107, CO_2 16

Homework problem #6

A dobutamine echo has an assumed sensitivity of 90% and specificity of 90% for detecting significant coronary artery disease. You are considering using the test to screen military pilots. The prevalence of CAD in this population is 5%.

- What % of patients testing positive will actually have the disease?
- What % of patients with normal results will *not* have CAD?

CHAPTER 3

Cardiology

Long QT syndrome (LQTS)

- LQTS is currently under-diagnosed.
- Because of this, it is over-represented on the Boards.
- Frequency is 1 in 3,000–5,000 individuals.
- Electrocardiogram (ECG) shows a prolongation of the QT interval.
- Propensity to ventricular tachyarrhythmias.
- May lead to syncope, cardiac arrest, or sudden death.
- QTc values usually above 0.46 seconds.

LQTS associations

- Romano-Ward syndrome (familial occurrence with autosomal dominant inheritance, QT prolongation, and ventricular tachyarrhythmias).
- Jervell and Lang-Nielsen (JLN) syndrome (familial occurrence with autosomal recessive inheritance, congenital deafness, QT prolongation, and ventricular arrhythmias).

LQTS presentation

- LQTS predisposes to *torsade de pointes* (polymorphic ventricular tachycardia) in otherwise healthy individuals.
- *Torsade de pointes* in patients with LQTS usually self-terminates.
- History may show a sudden cardiac death in a close family member.
- Cardiac event can be triggered by exercise (e.g., swimming), emotion, loud noise, or sleep.

LQTS treatment

- Beta blockers effective.
- Implantable cardioverter-defibrillators are an option for high-risk patients.
- Left cervicothoracic stellectomy is an alternative, antiadrenergic therapy in high-risk, refractory LQTS.
- Discourage these patients from participating in competitive sports.

Miscellaneous cardiac "pathognomonisms"

- *Parvus et Tardus* pulses: aortic stenosis.
- *Parvus* only: low output cardiomyopathy.
- Bifid pulse: Hypertrophic cardiomyopathy (from midsystolic obstruction).
- Fixed, split S_2 heart sound: atrial-septal defect.
- Opening snap: mitral stenosis.
- Continuous machinery murmur: patent *ductus arteriosus*.
- *Pulsus paradoxus* = cardiac tamponade.

Cardiac associations

- Marfan syndrome: dilatated aortic root.
- Syphilis: aortic regurgitation.
- Rheumatic heart disease: mitral stenosis.
- Maternal rubella: patent *ductus arteriosus*.

Valsalva effects

- Valsalva questions are common on the Board, despite being used rarely in practice.
- Valsalva maneuver decreases ventricular filling and decreases cardiac output.
- Thus, Valsalva effect serves to decrease the intensity of most murmurs . . . that is, *except* in the cases of those murmurs associated with hypertrophic cardiomyopathy and mitral valve prolapse.
- You must know these two exceptions to the Valsalva rule!

Drugs to avoid in pregnancy

- Captopril: fetal renal dysgenesis.
- Phenytoin: teratogenic.

- Warfarin: teratogenic, especially in first and third trimesters.
- While we're on the subject, a non-cardiac drug to avoid is tetracycline (it stains fetal teeth).

Cardiac tamponade signs

- Beck triad (jugular venous distention, hypotension, and muffled heart sounds).
- *Pulsus paradoxus* >10 mm Hg.
- "Triple pressures" equal on Swan.
- Electrical alternans.

Constrictive pericarditis signs

- Right-sided failure: peripheral edema, ascites, dyspnea, and fatigue.
- Kussmaul sign: inspiratory distention of neck veins.
- Pericardial knock.
- Square root sign on ventricular pressure curve.

Hemochromatosis

- Tetrad of liver disease, diabetes, brown skin, and congestive heart failure (CHF).
- Serum ferritin levels are high.
- Causes CHF and arrhythmias.
- Often presents with arthralgias, loss of libido, small gonads, and diabetes mellitus.

Cardiac drug side effects

- Procainamide: lupus-like syndrome.
- Lidocaine: seizure.
- Amiodarone: corneal deposits, photosensitivity, pulmonary fibrosis, increased liver function tests (LFTs), decreased warfarin clearance, and hypo- and hyperthyroidism.

Common reasons for pacing

- Symptomatic bradycardia due to any cause.
- Bradycardia from second or third degree heart block.
- Sinus node dysfunction.
- Carotid sinus hypersensitivity.

Reasons to pace an asymptomatic patient

- Consider pacing asymptomatic patients with these conditions:
  - Complete heart block.
  - Post-op AV block, after valve surgery, that does not resolve.
  - Mobitz II AV block

What is Mobitz II AV block?

- Defined as a sudden failure of P waves to conduct QRS waves.
- Shows constant PR intervals until a P wave occurs with no subsequent QRS.

Papillary muscle rupture

- Typically occurs 2–10 days after inferior or lateral myocardial infarction (MI).
- Typical case: a patient has been doing well post-MI, is recovering well on the wards, then suddenly develops dyspnea and hypotension.
- Diagnose with emergency echo.
- Treat with emergency surgery (balloon pump is next best choice).
- Loud murmur and thrill mean rupture with ventricular septal defect, but work-up and treatment are similar.

ECG in acute myocardial infarction

- Look for ST-segment elevation greater than one millimeter in two contiguous leads.
- May show new Q waves.
- ST-segment depression or T-wave inversion may indicate either ischemia or acute myocardial infarction.

Acute MI: distribution of ECG abnormalities

- Anteroseptal MI: abnormalities in V_1–V_3.
- Anterolateral MI: abnormalities in V_1–V_6.
- Inferior wall MI: abnormalities in II, III, aVF.
- Lateral wall MI: abnormalities in I, aVL, V_4–V_6.
- Right ventricular MI: abnormalities in RV_4, RV_5.
- Posterior wall MI: tall R-waves in V_1 and V_2 (R/S ratio greater than 1.0 in V_1 and V_2).

Progression of ECG findings in acute myocardial infarction

- Hyperacute T-waves may occur first.
- ST elevation occurs next.
- Q waves occur last.

Aortic stenosis

- Patients may remain asymptomatic until stenosis is severe.
- In severe cases, patients cannot increase cardiac output to meet increased demands of exercise or stress.
- The appearance of symptoms usually marks the beginning of a rapid downhill course.
- Dyspnea on exertion is the usual presenting complaint.
- Development of syncope, angina, or CHF indicates poor prognosis.

Aortic stenosis: murmur

- Systolic, crescendo-decrescendo murmur.
- Heard best at second intercostal space in the right upper sternal border.
- Harsh, rasping quality.
- Radiates to both carotid arteries.
- Late peaking murmurs of longer duration indicate more critical stenosis.

Mitral regurgitation

- Acute mitral regurgitation may present with orthopnea and pulmonary edema (e.g., inferior MI with papillary muscle dysfunction).
- Chronic mitral regurgitation may present with dyspnea on exertion or atrial fibrillation.
- The murmur of mitral regurgitation is apical and holosystolic.
- With acute mitral regurgitation, the murmur is harsh and may radiate across the entire precordium; may have thrill at apex.
- With chronic mitral regurgitation, the murmur radiates to the axilla.

Aortic regurgitation

- Patients with chronic aortic regurgitation show signs of left ventricle volume overload.
- Patients often remain asymptomatic for a long time period, then deteriorate rapidly after symptoms occur.

- Advanced cases present with dyspnea on exertion, orthopnea, and paroxysmal nocturnal dyspnea.
- De Musset sign: head bobs with each heartbeat.
- Corrigan pulse: water-hammer or collapsing pulse with rapid distention and then collapse.
- Pulse pressure may be greatly widened.
- May hear a decrescendo, diastolic murmur loudest at second- to fourth-left intercostal space adjacent to the sternum.

Mitral stenosis

- Most commonly presents 10–20 years after rheumatic fever.
- Patients may present with fatigue, dyspnea on exertion, chest pain, hemoptysis, or thromboembolism.
- May have diastolic thrill over apex.
- Loud S_1 and an S_2 opening snap heard best at sternal border.
- Murmur is low-pitched, rumbling, and diastolic; heard best over apex while patient is in the left lateral decubitus position.
- Duration of murmur correlates with severity.

Overview of supraventricular tachycardias (SVT)

- SVT is a narrow-complex tachycardia with regular rhythm; often caused by AV nodal re-entry; may be paroxysmal.
- Sinus tachycardia may be a normal physiological response or may be inappropriate (exaggerated sinus node response to autonomic stimuli).
- Multi-focal atrial tachycardia has P-waves with at least three different morphologies (usually elderly patients with pulmonary disorders); rhythm may be irregular (distinguish from atrial fibrillation).
- Atrial fibrillation has atrial rate of 300–600 and ventricular rate as high as 170 or greater; rhythm is irregularly irregular.
- Atrial flutter has an atrial rate of 250–350 beats per minute and a ventricular rate of approximately 150 beats per minute; usually 2:1 conduction; may see sawtooth flutter waves.

Paroxysmal supraventricular tachycardia (PSVT) treatment

- Can try vagal maneuvers (e.g., Valsalva) or carotid massage (unilateral) in stable patients with no bruits.
- Use synchronized cardioversion for unstable patients.

- Medical therapy: adenosine or calcium channel blockers; beta blockers for rate control.
- Radiofrequency ablation.

Wolff-Parkinson-White syndrome

- Usually cases are young, healthy patients; men affected more than women.
- Classically, baseline ECG shows short PR interval, wide QRS complex, and delta wave (slurred upstroke of QRS complex).
- Patients present with acute symptoms of tachycardia and symptoms of syncope, chest pain, and diaphoresis.
- Refer for radiofrequency ablation when stable.

Atrial fibrillation (AF)

- Irregularly irregular rhythm.
- Lack of P waves.
- If patient is stable, attempt to control ventricular rate with calcium channel blockers or beta blockers.
- Screen for causes including acute MI, pulmonary embolism, pneumonia, and hyperthyroidism.
- Anticoagulate for at least three weeks before attempting cardioversion.
- If AF is of unknown or greater than two days duration, screen patient with a trans-esophageal echocardiogram. If there is no thrombus seen in left atrium or right atrium, then okay to perform immediate electrical cardioversion. The patient still needs anticoagulation.

Atrial flutter

- Atrial rate 250–350 beats per minute.
- Can show sawtooth pattern in II, III, aVF.
- Generally a 2:1 or greater AV block.
- Ventricular rate is difficult to control, but AV nodal blockers (ibutilide, procainamide) can prevent 1:1 conduction.
- Patients require anticoagulation as with AF.

Multi-focal atrial tachycardia

- Rate 110–150 beats per minute.
- P waves show variable morphology.

- Most often 1:1 conduction.
- Results from sinus node dysfunction, theophylline, catecholamines, or severe illness.
- Treatment of underlying illness is most important.

Nonparoxysmal junctional tachycardia

- Rate 60–150 beats per minute.
- Normal QRS with either ventricular-atrial conduction or block with dissociation.
- Results from drugs, catecholamines, early post-op, or post-cardioversion.
- Treat with atrial pacing or ablation.

Treatment of sustained ventricular tachyarrhythmias

- For unstable ventricular tachycardia or ventricular fibrillation, cardioversion/defibrillation are the initial choices.
- For stable ventricular tachycardia, antiarrhythmic drugs are the initial choice to stabilize patients.
- However, long-term suppression of ventricular arrhythmias with class I or class III drugs has not shown survival benefit (and may even increase mortality).
- Both beta blockers and angiotensin converting enzyme inhibitors (ACE-Is) have shown a long-term survival benefit.
- Optimal treatment is an implantable cardioverter-defibrillator (ICD).

Treatment of unstable angina

- Admit to coronary care unit to rule out acute MI.
- Beta blockers and IV nitroglycerin if tolerated; oxygen if needed.
- Aspirin and heparin (including low-molecular-weight heparin).
- Glycoprotein Iib/IIIa inhibitors.
- Cardiology consult for cardiac catheterization (urgently, if symptoms do not abate).

Miscellaneous cardiology pearls

- Use calcium gluconate for hyperkalemia with ECG changes.
- For pre-operative evaluation, the finding of an S_3 heart sound is the highest single predictor of cardiovascular risk.

- Post-MI patients need aspirin and beta blockers.
- Use ACE inhibitors in patients with CHF; alternative is minoxidil and hydralazine combination, especially in African American patients.

Bacterial endocarditis

- Treat penicillin-sensitive, *Streptococcus* native valve endocarditis with penicillin with gentamicin for two weeks.
- Treat *Enterococcus* native valve endocarditis with penicillin with gentamicin for four weeks.
- Treat *Staphylococcus aureus* native valve endocarditis with gentamicin and penicillin for four weeks (substitute vancomycin if penicillin resistant).
- For prosthetic valves, treat methicillin-resistant *Staphylococcus* with vancomycin and rifampin for four weeks; for first two weeks, include gentamicin as well.

Coarctation of the aorta

- A narrowing of the aortic lumen that obstructs blood flow.
- Increased afterload can lead to hypertension and left ventricular hypertrophy; CHF may be present.
- Dilation of intercostal artery collaterals can lead to rib notching on chest radiography.
- Look for a blood pressure gradient between arms and legs.
- Lower extremity pulses may be diminished.

Takayasu arteritis

- A chronic, inflammatory, occlusive disease of the aorta and its branches.
- More frequently seen in Asian or Indian patients.
- Systolic blood pressure difference is typically greater than 10 mm Hg between arms.
- Constitutional symptoms are common (fever, weight loss, and malaise).
- Distal pulses are typically absent or diminished pulses, but may be bounding as well (unlike coarctation).

Medical treatment of acute cardiac ischemia (without ST elevation on ECG)

- Oxygen if O_2 saturation is less than 90%.
- Aspirin.

- Beta blockers (contraindicated in high-grade AV block).
- Heparin or low-molecular-weight heparin.
- Angiotensin converting enzyme inhibitor if hypertensive or signs of LV dysfunction.
- Nitroglycerin and morphine for ongoing pain.
- Use glycoprotein IIb/IIIa inhibitors in patients who are likely to need percutaneous intervention.
- Proceed to percutaneous intervention for refractory chest pain or hypotension.

Treatment of acute myocardial infarction (ST elevation or new LBBB on ECG)

- Treat as in acute cardiac ischemia above.
- In addition, consider fibrinolytic therapy (e.g., t-PA) if ST elevation >2 mm in at least two contiguous leads, if patient is under 75 years old, and if within 12 hours of symptom onset.
- Percutaneous intervention, if immediately available, is preferred to fibrinolytic therapy.

CHAPTER 4

Gastroenterology

Zollinger-Ellison syndrome

- Presents with triad of peptic ulcer, acid hypersecretion, and diarrhea.
- Results from gastrin-producing tumor in the pancreas or duodenum.
- Suspect this in any patient with unusual or unexplained duodenal ulcer.
- Diagnose with gastrin level >1,000 pg/mL.
- Localize tumor with Octreotide scan.
- Note: Octreotide is a somatostatin analogue.

Somatostatinoma

- Results in overproduction of somatostatin from delta cells of pancreas.
- Somatostatin stimulates gastric emptying, but inhibits most other biliary and pancreas secretions.
- Clinical result of this wide inhibition effect is steatorrhea, weight loss, cholelithiasis, and diabetes.
- Seven percent of cases are associated with MEN1 syndrome.
- Treat with surgery or chemotherapy based on 5-FU.

VIPoma

- Vasoactive intestinal peptide (VIP) is also secreted by delta cells of pancreas.
- Tumor results in copious, watery diarrhea, dehydration, and flushing.
- Lab shows hypokalemia and non-gap acidosis (from bicarb wasting).
- Control symptoms with somatostatin.

Carcinoid syndrome

- Symptoms produced by metastases of carcinoid tumors.
- Clinical: flushing, diarrhea, hypotension, hyperthermia, and tachycardia.
- Screen with urinary 5-HIAA level.
- Most tumors located in terminal ileum; however, symptoms do not occur until they metastasize to liver.
- Treat symptoms with somatostatin analogue (Octreotide).

Bacterial overgrowth

- Suspect bacterial overgrowth in any patient with diarrhea and macrocytic anemia.
- Bacteria cause deconjugation of bile acids.
- As a result, bile acids are absorbed early in duodenum.
- This leads to steatorrhea of 10–20 g per day.
- Patients also get B_{12} deficiency.
- Folate level is increased (from bacterial production).

Celiac sprue

- Suspect when you have iron deficiency with negative work up for blood loss, which is *not* responsive to iron therapy.
- Response to a gluten-free diet strongly suggests diagnosis.
- Gold standard for diagnosis is small bowel biopsy.
- Clinical: steatorrhea, gastrointestinal (GI) upset, and growth retardation.
- Patients may have associated dermatitis herpetiformis.

Tropical sprue

- Look for history of travel to tropics in the previous 3–6 months.
- Clinical: diarrhea and megaloblastic anemia (from folate deficiency).
- Caused by *Klebsiella* and *Escherichia coli*.
- Treat with tetracycline and folate.

Secretory diarrhea

- Larger stool volume than in osmotic diarrhea (usually greater than one L/day).
- Increased loss of electrolytes.
- Examples are cholera, *E. coli* enterotoxins.

Osmotic diarrhea

- Smaller stool volume than in secretory diarrhea (usually less than one L/day).
- Osmotic gap due to a non-absorbable substance.
- Causes: lactase deficiency, sorbitol, antacids, etc.

Enterotoxigenic diarrhea

- Also known as "traveler's diarrhea."
  - Usually from enterotoxigenic strain of *E. coli.*
  - Stool typically has no blood or white blood cells (WBCs).
  - Large volume diarrhea; treat with fluid replacement.
  - Treat with antibiotics (e.g., ciprofloxacin) only if febrile.

Invasive diarrhea

- Caused by *Campylobacter, Shigella, Salmonella, E. coli* strain 0157:H7, etc.
- Stool often shows blood and WBCs.
- Patients may show signs of systemic infection (e.g., fever).

Clostridium difficile

- Causes an antibiotic-associated, pseudomembranous colitis.
- Onset is one week after antibiotic started, or up to eight weeks after antibiotics are stopped.
- Patients usually have WBCs in stool.
- Treatment is to stop the antibiotic and give metronidazole.
- If treatment fails, give metronidazole again (yes, repeat the same treatment with metronidazole for the same duration).
- Consider vancomycin for refractory cases.

Meckel diverticulum

- A congenital GI anomaly leading to GI bleed, obstruction, or intussusception.
- Most likely choice for lower GI bleed in child or young adult.
- Screen with technetium scan.

Familial polyposis

- Typical Board question: patient has multiple family members with history of colon cancer.

- Colonoscopy shows extensive adenomatous polyps.
- "Refer for colectomy" is usually the correct answer.

Stage C colon cancer

- A very common Board question.
- Stage C = (tumor penetrates into and/or through the muscularis propria of bowel wall) + (pathologic evidence of colon cancer in lymph nodes).
- Treatment is with 5-fluorouracil and leukovorin.

Primary biliary cirrhosis

- Usually middle-aged women.
- Clinical: pruritis and fatigue.
- Increased alkaline phosphatase on lab.
- The clue: elevated antimitochondrial antibodies (AMA).
- Treat with ursodiol.

Primary sclerosing cholangitis

- An autoimmune fibrosis of large bile ducts.
- Clinical: right upper quadrant abdominal pain, fatigue, and weight loss.
- Seventy percent of cases associated with ulcerative colitis.
- Associated with an increased risk of cholangiocarcinoma.
- Diagnose with ERCP.

Whipple disease

- A relapsing, slowly progressive, systemic infectious disease.
- Clinical: fever, polyarthralgia, and diarrhea.
- May cause culture-negative endocarditis and thromboembolism.
- Causative organism: *Tropheryma whippelli*.
- Diagnose with biopsy of involved organ.
- Antibiotic treatment: induction with ceftriaxone for two to four weeks, then TMP-SMX for one to two years.

Wilson disease

- Total bilirubin/direct bilirubin ratio increased on lab.
- Clinical: altered mental status.
- Kayser-Fleischer ring: brown ring at periphery of cornea (from copper).

- Screen by drawing lab to look for low ceruloplasmin level.
- Confirm with liver biopsy.
- Treat with penicillamine or liver transplant.

Gilbert syndrome

- The leading cause of elevated indirect bilirubin.
- Also the leading cause of hyperbilirubinemia.
- Usually found incidentally on metabolic panel.
- Gilbert syndrome is a benign condition present in 5% of the population.

Ascites evaluation

- First determine whether it is high-grade ascites (i.e., transudate) versus low-grade ascites (i.e., exudate).
- Determine serum-to-ascites albumin gradient (the difference between the two values).
- If serum-ascites albumin gradient >1.1, you have high-grade ascites (e.g., cirrhosis, congestive heart failure [CHF], portal vein thrombosis).
- If serum-ascites albumin gradient >1.1, you have low-grade ascites (e.g., pancreatitis, tuberculosis, etc.).

Dysphagia evaluation

- Perform barium swallow first (before endoscopy).
- Perform endoscopy next.
- Motility studies if above tests negative or inconclusive.

Squamous cell carcinoma of the esophagus

- Predisposing conditions include the following:
  - Achalasia.
  - Lye stricture.
  - Plummer-Vinson syndrome.
  - Human papilloma virus.
  - Alcohol and tobacco use.
  - Tylosis.

Achalasia

- A failure of the hypertensive, lower esophageal sphincter to relax, combined with an absence of esophageal peristalsis.

- Clinical: dysphagia, regurgitation, chest pain, heartburn, and weight loss.
- Key radiographic finding is smooth, beaklike tapering on upper GI.
- Treatment is pneumatic dilatation by a qualified gastroenterologist.

Plummer-Vinson syndrome

- Triad of dysphagia, upper esophageal webs, and iron deficiency anemia.
- Dysphagia is intermittent and usually limited to solids.
- Dysphagia improves after iron therapy.
- Weakness, fatigue, and dyspnea are frequent complaints (symptoms respond to iron replacement).

Tylosis

- Esophageal papillomas + hyperkeratosis of the palms and soles.
- A rare, autosomal dominant disorder.

Diffuse esophageal spasm

- Hallmark is chest pain.
- Unlike achalasia, diffuse esophageal spasm has normal relaxation intermittently.
- Barium swallow may show "corkscrew" esophagus.

Barrett esophagus

- Characterized by finding specialized intestinal metaplasia in the esophagus.
- Is a complication of gastroesophageal reflux disease (GERD).
- Risk for development of adenocarcinoma in the esophagus.
- Diagnose with EGD and biopsy (not barium swallow).

Zenker diverticulum

- Caused by an esophageal mucosa herniation; thus Zenker's is a "pseudo"-diverticulum.
- The diverticulum will retain food in its pouch.
- Leads to halitosis, regurgitation, aspiration, and dysphagia.
- Managed by surgical repair.

Spontaneous bacterial peritonitis

- Clinical: fever and abdominal tenderness in a patient with ascites.
- Lab: WBC usually greater than 500 on paracentesis.
- Diagnosis requires high index of suspicion.
- Treat with third generation cephalosporin to cover enterobacteriaceae, streptococcus pneumoniae, and enterococci.

Boerhaave syndrome

- Esophageal perforation, usually from retching.
- Results from alcoholism, or may be iatrogenic (e.g., can occur after dilatation of esophageal strictures).
- Gastrograffin (water soluble contrast) reveals location of extravasation.
- Treat with surgical repair of esophagus, debridement of mediastinum, and pleural drainage.

Esophageal varices

- Nonselective beta blocker (e.g., propranolol) is best prophylaxis to prevent initial bleed.
- Band ligation for long-term management of hemorrhage.
- Transjugular intrahepatic portosystemic shunt (TIPS) procedure only if banding fails to control hemorrhage.

Angiodysplasia

- A vascular ecstasia of the GI tract.
- Causes painless lower GI bleeding.
- Most common in elderly.

Acute mesenteric ischemia

- Only 50% of cases are related to thrombus or embolus.
- The other half are non-occlusive, such as from a low-flow state associated with hypotension or vasospasm.
- Clinical: may show abdominal pain with relatively benign abdominal exam.
- Very ill patients will have an elevated anion gap metabolic acidosis.
- Order angiography and immediate surgery consultation.

Chronic mesenteric ischemia

- Clinical: abdominal pain after meals, weight loss, and abdominal bruit.
- Results from chronic occlusion of splanchnic arteries.
- Diagnose with angiography.

Irritable bowel syndrome

- Functional GI disorder causing pain and abnormal bowel habits.
- A diagnosis of exclusion.
- Abdominal pain is relieved by defecation, or may be associated with a change in stool frequency or consistency.
- Symptoms may improve or resolve with avoidance of stress, along with successful treatment of underlying psychological disorders.

Viral hepatitis: transmission

- Fecal-oral route: Hepatitis A and E.
- Sexual route: Hepatitis B and D; and to a lesser extent C.
- Parenteral route: Hepatitis B, C, and D; and to a lesser extent A.
- Note: Hepatitis D requires coexisting Hepatitis B infection.

Viral hepatitis: clinical

- Symptoms include fatigue, anorexia, nausea, and vomiting.
- Lab shows elevated AST, ALT, and bilirubin.
- Course may resolve, may turn fulminant, or may become chronic.

Hepatitis A

- Common in the Middle East, Africa, Asia, and Latin countries.
- Incubation period 15–45 days.
- Children are often asymptomatic.
- Treatment is supportive.
- IgG anti-HepA indicates previous exposure and thus lifelong immunity.
- Hepatitis A vaccine given in two or three parts.
- Immune globulin for travel up to three months in endemic area or for close contacts of cases.

Hepatitis B

- Five percent of world's population has chronic Hepatitis B (defined by positive HBsAg).

- Five percent of adults with acute HBV go on to develop chronic infection.
- Twenty percent of chronic cases progress to cirrhosis or hepatocellular carcinoma.
- Average incubation period is 12 weeks.

Hepatitis B serology

- HBsAg does not indicate whether the infection is acute versus chronic.
- IgM anti-HBc = acute HBV infection.
- Total anti-HBc (IgM and IgG) indicates a history of HBV infection at some point.
- Anti-HBsAb titers rise as infection clears.
- HBeAg is a marker for high HBV DNA levels and active replication.
- After the vaccine series, 95% develop the anti-HBsAb marker.

Hepatitis C

- Average incubation period is eight weeks.
- Condom is not currently part of recommendations if the patient has a steady partner, but they should not share razors or toothbrush.
- Interferon is the mainstay of treatment for chronic infection, but has a very high incidence of serious side effects.

Hepatitis D

- Cannot replicate by itself; requires co-existing hepatitis B infection.
- Superinfection may cause an apparent worsening or flare of hepatitis B cases.
- Increases risk of fulminant progression.

Hepatitis E

- Enterically transmitted.
- Clinical picture is similar to hepatitis A.
- Treatment is supportive.
- May cause fulminant hepatitis if a pregnant woman acquires it in her third trimester.

Acute pancreatitis

- Causes: alcohol abuse, gallstones, medications, etc.
- Screen for pancreatic necrosis with CT scan.

- Use antibiotic treatment (imipenem, cefuroxime) for necrosis or for severe pancreatitis with organ failure.

Pancreatic cancer

- Extremely aggressive with poor prognosis.
- Clinical: jaundice, weight loss, abdominal pain, or mass.
- Associated with tumor marker CA 19-9.
- Treat with resection (Whipple procedure) if tumor is in head of pancreas, and if no metastasis is suspected.

Inflammatory bowel disease (IBD)

- An idiopathic, immune reaction of the body against its own GI tract.
- Ulcerative colitis (UC), as its name implies, is limited to the colon.
- Crohn disease involves any part of the GI tract, from mouth to anus.

Colon cancer risk in IBD

- Colon cancer risk in UC begins to rise 8–10 years after diagnosis.
- Surveillance colonoscopy with random biopsy reduces mortality in patients with UC (due to early diagnosis).
- Crohn disease, if it involves the entire colon, is now thought to have a risk ratio for colon cancer equal to UC.

IBD: clinical

- Ulcerative colitis: most often bloody diarrhea.
- Crohn disease: diarrhea and pain.
- Both have anemia and fatigue.
- Ulcerative colitis: risk for toxic megacolon.
- Crohn disease: fistulae, strictures, and obstructions; affects entire intestinal wall, unlike UC (which is mucosa only).

Treatment of IBD

- First step: aminosalicylates.
- Second step: corticosteroids.
- Third step: immunomodulatory medications.
  - Examples: 6-MP, azathioprine.
  - Requires close monitoring of labs.

- Another option is infliximab, a monoclonal antibody against tumor necrosis factor alpha.
- Surgery reserved for strictures, etc. and dysplasia on biopsy or if symptoms are refractory.

Diverticulitis

- Clinical: left lower quadrant abdominal pain and tenderness, fever, high WBC count.
- For severe symptoms, screen with CT scan to rule out abscess.
- Outpatient treatment: metronidazole + ciprofloxacin.

CHAPTER 5

Pulmonology and Critical Care

Horner syndrome

- Ipsilateral *miosis* (constricted pupil), *anhidrosis* (absence of sweating), and *ptosis* (partially failed eyelid opening) on the side of the lesion.
- Seen with Pancoast tumor (superior sulcus tumor of lung).
- Often squamous cell carcinomas.

Obligatory asthma question

- Correct answer for a moderately severe, acute outpatient flare is usually to add oral prednisone (if patient already on β_2 agonist inhalers).
- Correct answer for chronic treatment is usually to add inhaled steroid to β_2 agonist inhalers.

Cystic fibrosis: background

- Highly prevalent on Boards.
- Many patients undiagnosed until young adulthood.
- Autosomal recessive (know this).
- Allergic bronchopulmonary aspergillosis often seen in cystic fibrosis (CF) patients.

Cystic fibrosis: diagnosis

- Need high index of suspicion.
- Check for abnormally high sweat chloride levels (greater than 80 mEq/L in adult).

- Diagnosis also based on finding clinical symptoms of CF, positive family history, and signs of pancreatic insufficiency.

Cystic fibrosis: associations

- Sinusitis and nasal polyposis.
- Hemoptysis.
- Pneumothorax.
- Pancreatic insufficiency.
- Chronic obstructive pulmonary disease (COPD) is invariably present in adults with CF and is the major cause of mortality.

Cystic fibrosis: prognosis

- Patients are now living longer thanks to improved recognition and treatment of infections.
- More than 50% survive past the age of 25.
- Key to survival is good chest physical therapy, aggressive nutrition, and avoidance of cold climates.
- Need to treat respiratory infections early with broad-spectrum antibiotics.

Bronchiectasis

- Defined as an ectasia of the bronchi due to destruction of bronchial walls.
- Seen with pneumonia, chronic bronchitis, allergic bronchopulmonary aspergillosis, and CF.
- Patients have anorexia, weight loss, fetor oris (foul breath), and arthralgia.
- Diagnose with high-resolution CT (shows "signet-ring" shadows).

Kartagener syndrome

- A rare cause of bronchiectasis (<1%).
- It is an inherited triad of situs inversus, sinusitis, and bronchiectasis.
- Basic defect is immotile cilia.
- Kartagener syndrome is a common cause of dextrocardia.

Allergic bronchopulmonary aspergillosis: diagnostic criteria

- Asthma.
- Blood eosinophilia above 1×10^9/L.
- Type I (IgE) immediate skin reaction to *Aspergillus*.
- IgG (type III) reaction to *Aspergillus*.
- IgE >1000 ng/ML. (This test should be ordered.)
- Pulmonary infiltrates are often fleeting.
- Central bronchiectasis.
- Note: treat with long-term prednisone (6–12 months).

Bronchiolitis obliterans with organizing pneumonia (BOOP)

- Patients present with signs and symptoms of a very prolonged respiratory infection.
- May develop after prolonged viral and bacterial infections, radiation therapy, collagen vascular disease, or toxin exposure.
- Screen with high-resolution chest CT; may need to confirm with lung biopsy.
- Treat confirmed cases with corticosteroids.

Interpreting pleural fluid

- Transudate = serum to effusion albumin gradient >1.2 g/dL and protein content <3g.
- Transudate often results from congestive heart failure (CHF) although there is a long differential diagnosis.
- Exudate often results from pneumonia.
- Finding of elevated amylase in pleural fluid could mean pancreatitis or esophageal rupture.
- Low complement and high ANA levels could mean systemic lupus erythematosus.
- High adenosine deaminase and interferon-gamma levels are a clue to a tuberculous effusion.

Wegener granulomatosis: background

- A necrotizing, granulomatous vasculitis.
- Involves upper and lower respiratory tract.

- Usually presents along with glomerulonephritis.
- Characterized by variable, small-vessel vasculitis.
- More than 90% of patients are white; average age is 45.

Wegener granulomatosis: presentation

- Upper respiratory tract signs: sinus pain and/or drainage, mucosal ulcerations, epistaxis, otalgia, and otitis media.
- Lower respiratory tract signs: cough, dyspnea, and hemoptysis (may be massive).
- Screen with cytoplasmic-antineutrophil cytoplasmic antibody (c-ANCA).

Wegener granulomatosis: treatment

- Treat with corticosteroids and cyclophosphamide.
- Methotrexate and azathioprine are alternatives to maintain remission.

Sarcoidosis

- Often young patients with erythema nodosum, arthritis, abnormal CXR, and fever.
- Serum ACE levels are not sensitive or specific, and are usually the wrong answer.
- Bronchoscopy with biopsy (to look for non-caseating granulomas) is the best diagnostic test if adenopathy and hilar infiltrates are present.
- Treat with corticosteroids.

Histiocytosis X

- An uncommon disease of young, white men who smoke.
- Characterized by abnormal infiltration of the lungs with Langerhans cells (>5%).
- Clinical: spontaneous pneumothorax, dry cough, dyspnea, chest pain, fatigue, and fever.
- May also have painful, cystic bone lesions.
- May have central nervous system (CNS) involvement (e.g., central diabetes insipidus).
- Treatment is mandatory smoking cessation.

Asbestosis

- Presents 15–30 years after exposure.
- Clinical: dyspnea, crackles, and restriction on pulmonary function tests (PFTs).
- CXR and CT may show effusions, rounded atelectasis, interstitial changes, volume loss, and pleural thickening.
- Malignant mesotheliomas are highly related to asbestos exposure, but are unrelated to smoking.

Silicosis

- From inhalation of crystalline silica (e.g., sandblasting, quarrying, mining, or grinding and polishing of stone).
- Clinical: progressive dyspnea and cough with rales; can progress to *cor pulmonale* and respiratory failure.
- Higher incidence of *mycobacterial* diseases in patients with silicosis.
- Chest radiography may show simple nodules, ground glass appearance, or "eggshell" hilar node calcification.
- Patients should have annual TB screening with PPD skin test.

Lung neoplasm pearls

- Squamous cell carcinoma often arises in proximal airway.
- Adenocarcinoma often arises in periphery.
- Bronchoalveolar cell carcinoma risk is unrelated to cigarette smoking.
- Small cell cancer leads to paraneoplastic syndromes (SIADH, ACTH, myasthenic syndrome); look for abnormal CXR and weakness, hypokalemia, or hypercalcemia.

Positive PPD criteria

- Greater than or equal to 5 mm: for high-risk patients (HIV, close contact with infectious case, or fibrotic CXR changes).
- Greater than or equal to 10 mm: at-risk patients (e.g., healthcare workers, nursing home residents).
- Greater than or equal to 15 mm: if no risk factors for TB.

Recent PPD converter criteria

- Greater than or equal to 10 mm change in 2 years (age <35).
- Greater than or equal to 15 mm change in 2 years (age ≥35).

Side effects of tuberculosis drugs

- Isoniazid: hepatitis and peripheral neuropathy.
- Rifampin: gastrointestincal upset; increased metabolism of warfarin.
- Pyrazinamide: liver toxicity.
- Ethambutol: dose-related retrobulbar neuritis (worse in renal insufficiency).

Obstructive sleep apnea

- Patients may report morning headache, daytime drowsiness, and history of snoring.
- Clinical: may see hypertension, peripheral edema, and polycythemia.
- Treat with nasal CPAP.

Criteria for initiating 24-hour nasal O_2 in COPD outpatients

- Patient has resting P_aO_2 less than 55, or
- O_2 saturation less than 89%, or
- O_2 saturation greater than 88% with evidence of *cor pulmonale*.

Idiopathic pulmonary fibrosis (IPF)

- A chronic, progressive lung disease of unknown origin.
- Clinical: progressive dyspnea on exertion, interstitial infiltrates on chest radiograph, and restrictive pattern on pulmonary function tests.
- Patients have expiratory "velcro" rales in lung bases.
- Diagnose with open lung biopsy to exclude other diseases.
- Treat with corticosteroids.

Primary pulmonary hypertension

- An idiopathic, increased pulmonary artery pressure leads to arteriopathy and micro-thrombosis of pulmonary vasculature.
- Clinical: dyspnea; increased pulmonic component of the second heart sound.
- Female predominance; rare.
- Exposure to stimulant drugs may increase risk.
- Treatment is anticoagulation with warfarin.
- Also treat associated right-sided heart failure and ascites if present.
- Lung transplant for refractory cases.

Alpha-1 antitrypsin deficiency

- Clinical: early-onset symptoms of COPD.
- Alpha-1 antitrypsin normally inhibits elastase, the destructive pulmonary enzyme.
- Disease is accelerated by cigarette smoking.
- Treat with pulmonary rehabilitation.
- Prolastin is a pooled, purified, human plasma protein concentrate replacement of alpha-1 antitrypsin; use weekly infusions.
- Consider lung transplantation.

Acute respiratory distress syndrome (ARDS)

- Noncardiac pulmonary edema and hypoxemic respiratory failure.
- Diagnosis requires: acute onset, bilateral pulmonary infiltrates, normal pulmonary artery wedge pressure, and persistently low PaO_2 despite high concentrations of supplemental oxygen.
- Very high mortality; patients who recover usually develop some degree of pulmonary fibrosis.
- On ventilator use tidal volume (V_t) of 6 ml/kg and adequate positive end-expiratory pressure (PEEP).

Mechanical ventilation: weaning criteria

- Patient is stable, alert, and appears strong; minimal secretions.
- Adequate tidal volume; respiratory rate less than 30.
- FiO_2 less than 40%.
- PaO_2 greater than 60 mm Hg.
- PEEP less than 5 mm Hg.
- Maximum inspiratory force should be less than −25 mm Hg (more negative is better).

Pneumococcal pneumonia in hospitalized patients

- Acceptable to treat with penicillin; cephalosporin if sensitive to penicillin.
- If resistant to penicillin, use fluoroquinolone such as levofoxacin or vancomycin.
- If meningitis is a concern, use vancomycin and ceftriaxone pending cultures (fluoroquinolones do not penetrate CNS well).

Community-acquired methicillin resistant Staphylococcus aureus (MRSA) infection

- MRSA incidence is increasing in community.
- Can cause extremely severe infection, including bacteremia, osteomyelitis, soft tissue infections, and urinary tract infections, and may require prolonged ICU care.
- MRSA pneumonia may cause extreme morbidity including shock, respiratory failure, disseminated intravascular coagulopathy (DIC), and limb necrosis requiring amputation.

Respiratory syncytial virus (RSV)

- Leading cause of lower respiratory tract infection in young children.
- By age three, nearly every child has had at least one RSV infection; in some cases requires hospitalization.
- Reinfection occurs at all ages; with increasing age and number of infections, RSV tends to be limited to upper respiratory tract.
- Prompt antivirus therapy with aerosolized ribavirin is indicated for high-risk patients.
- Adults at greatest risk include elderly and immunosuppressed.

Influenza

- Causes very high mortality in COPD patients.
- Treatment with amantadine or rimantadine is effective prophylaxis for influenza A.
- If given within first 24 hours of onset of illness, amantadine or rimantadine reduces severity and duration of influenza A infection.
- For outbreaks of influenza A in nursing homes, treat *everyone* in the nursing home with amantadine prophylaxis.
- If given early, oseltamivir and zanamivir reduce severity of both influenza A and influenza B infections.

Human metapneumovirus (hMPV)

- hMPV is a more recently identified virus of the Paramyxoviridae family.
- Clinically indistinguishable from RSV infection.
- Causes severe respiratory tract infection in children and adults over 65 years of age.

- Diagnose with Polymerase Chain Reaction (PCR) treatment is unknown.

Severe acute respiratory syndrome (SARS)

- The SARS-associated coronavirus (SARS-CoV) is a more recently recognized member of the Coronaviridae family.
- Coronaviridae were previously known simply as a major cause of the common cold.
- SARS-CoV may have originated from animals and spread to humans via close contact in rural, southern China.
- SARS includes a flu-like syndrome that may progress to pneumonia, respiratory failure, and death.
- In humans, SARS is transmitted by close human-to-human contact (including airplane travel).
- Overall mortality is 10%, with greater than 50% mortality in patients over age 65.
- Treatment is supportive, including critical care if respiratory function deteriorates.

Avian influenza (Bird flu)

- Carried by wild birds; cause morbidity in domestic birds.
- Influenza A virus strain H5N1 mutates rapidly.
- Strains of avian H5N1 influenza can infect many kinds of animals.
- Close contact with infected poultry has been the primary source of human infection.
- Symptoms in humans range from influenza-like symptoms to conjunctivitis, acute respiratory distress, and severe, viral pneumonia.
- H5N1 viruses are generally resistant to amantadine and rimantadine.
- Instead, treat with oseltamivir or zanamavir.

Superior vena cava syndrome

- A medical emergency caused by obstruction of blood flow through the superior vena cava.
- Obstruction usually due to malignancy; mostly bronchogenic carcinomas (especially small cell carcinoma).
- Immediate danger is from laryngeal and cerebral edema.
- Clinical: dyspnea, face or arm swelling, dysphagia, orthopnea, cough, chest pain, stridor, mental status changes, etc.
- Treat with head elevation, supplemental oxygen, and irradiation.

Pulmonary embolism (PE)

- Diagnosis of PE requires a high index of suspicion; it is one of the most frequently missed diagnoses.
- Risk factors include recent surgery, immobility, hypercoagulable state, pregnancy, oral contraceptives, estrogen, or selective estrogen receptor modifiers.
- Clinical: may show dyspnea, pleuritic chest pain, cough, and hemoptysis, but most patients with PE have no obvious symptoms.
- Most patients diagnosed with deep venous thrombosis (DVT) will also have asymptomatic pulmonary emboli.
- Screen for PE with V/Q perfusion scan or spiral CT of lungs; sensitivity can be increased by combining with ultrasound or CT to screen for DVT.
- Pulmonary angiography remains the gold standard for diagnosis.
- Treatment: For anyone suspected to have DVT or PE, immediately begin heparin or low-molecular-weight heparin; follow with warfarin.
- Consider thrombolytic therapy for patients who are hemodynamically unstable.
- Consider inferior vena cava filter if anticoagulation is absolutely contraindicated, for recurrent venous thromboembolism despite adequate anticoagulation, or for massive PE in which a recurrent embolism could be fatal.

Tension pneumothorax

- Injured tissue forms a one-way valve, trapping air in the pleural space.
- Progresses rapidly to respiratory failure, cardiovascular collapse, or death if not treated promptly.
- Common causes include external trauma, central venous line placement, or barotrauma from using high PEEP on mechanical ventilation.
- Early signs include chest pain, dyspnea, tachypnea, tachycardia; hyperresonance and diminished breath sounds on the affected side.
- On mechanically ventilated patients, suspect tension pneumothorax when increased pleural pressures require increased peak airway pressures in order to deliver the same tidal volume.
- Treat with urgent needle decompression, followed by placement of a thoracostomy tube.
- Perform needle decompression without hesitation: using a long, 14-gauge needle with catheter, puncture the second rib interspace at the midclavicular line.

CHAPTER 6

Rheumatology

Rheumatoid Arthritis (RA) diagnostic criteria (need 4 out of 7)

- One hour or greater morning stiffness.
- Three or more joints affected simultaneously.
- Wrist, metacarpophalangeal (MCP), or proximal interphalangeal joints (PIP) involved.
- Symmetrical arthritis.
- Rheumatoid nodules.
- Elevated serum rheumatoid factor.
- Typical X-ray changes (e.g., erosions, joint space narrowing).

Extra-articular manifestations of Rheumatoid Arthritis

- Cardiac: myocarditis, accelerated atherosclerosis.
- Neurologic: mononeuritis multiplex (foot or wrist drop).
- Hematologic: anemia of chronic disease, neutropenia, or vasculitis.
- Pulmonary: pulmonary nodules, interstitial fibrosis, or pleural effusion.
- Renal: amyloid.
- Skin: rheumatoid nodules.

Cervical spine involvement of Rheumatoid Arthritis

- Fifty percent of RA patients have cervical spine involvement.
- May present with neck pain, syncope, light-headedness, or paresthesias.

- Check cervical flexion and extension X-rays.
- Symptomatic patients require prompt intubation to maintain airway.

Side effects of rheumatology medications

- NSAIDs = bone marrow toxicity, tinnitus, pulmonary infiltrates, and renal papillary necrosis among many other side effects.
- Hydroxychloroquine = retinopathy.
- Gold = bone marrow suppression and rash.
- Methotrexate = gastrointestinal distress and bone marrow suppression (give folic acid supplement with methotrexate).
- Cyclophosphamide = neoplasia, hemorrhagic cystitis (but the toxic metabolite of cyclophosphamide, known as acrolein, can be neutralized by treatment with mesna).

Still disease

- A juvenile form of RA.
- Patients are seronegative for RA and antinuclear antibody (ANA).
- Quotidian fevers (spike and return to normal in same day).
- Macular, evanescent rash.
- Large joints affected.
- Sore throat is a common feature.

Felty syndrome

- Classic triad of RA, leukopenia, and splenomegaly.
- May also see recurrent fever, weight loss, lymphadenopathy, and vasculitis.

Baker Cyst

- Popliteal swelling in RA patients.
- May rupture and mimic deep venous thrombosis (DVT).
- Diagnose with ultrasound.
- Differential diagnosis = popliteal artery aneurysm, phlebitis, or tumor.

Pseudoclaudication

- Exertional calf or thigh cramping raises question of claudication.
- Symptoms improve when leaning forward.

- Key: check peripheral pulses; if normal, it is pseudoclaudication from spinal stenosis, rather than claudication.

Carpal tunnel syndrome

- Median nerve compression at the wrist causes ischemia and impaired axonal transport.
- Clinical: pain and paresthesias in the median nerve distribution of the hand (palmar and radial).
- Symptoms worse at night.
- Weakness and thenar atrophy occur later.
- Carpal tunnel syndrome is commonly associated with pregnancy, RA, and dialysis. These are common Board associations.

Temporal arteritis

- Age >50.
- Female:Male = 3:1.
- Most common in Northern Europeans.
- Clinical: temporal headache, fatigue, and fever.
- Very high sedimentation rate on lab tests.
- Treat with high dose prednisone, pending temporal artery biopsy, in order to prevent blindness.

Polyarteritis nodosa

- Systemic, necrotizing vasculitis.
- Clinical: fever, fatigue, weight loss, and myalgia.
- Kidneys and lungs are involved.
- Lab: normocytic anemia, high ESR, and thrombocytosis.
- p-ANCA often positive.
- A similar polyarteritis can occur with RA, systemic lupus erythematosus, cryoglobulinema, hepatitis B, and malignancy.
- Diagnosis: angiography or biopsy (shows vasculitis).

Churg-Strauss vasculitis

- Similar to polyarteritis, but more cardiac involvement.
- Typical patient has asthma, nasal polyposis, and palpable purpura.
- Diagnosis requires demonstrating:
  - Asthma.

- Eosinophilia ($>1.5 \times 10^9$ eos/L).
- Systemic vasculitis of two or more extrapulmonary organs.

Buerger disease

- Thromboangiitis obliterans.
- Seen only in young adult smokers.
- Digit ischemia leading to amputation.
- Usually resolves with smoking cessation.

Cryoglobulinemia

- Cryoglobulins are immunoglobulins that reversibly precipitate with cold (note: these are completely different from "cold agglutinins").
- Type I = leads to increased viscosity, thus causing headache, visual disturbances, and nosebleeds (associated with Waldenstrom macroglobulinemia, lymphoma).
- Type II = leads to palpable purpura, urticaria (associated with hepatitis C, autoimmune disorders, lymphoma).

Cryoglobulinemia: lab diagnosis

- High sedimentation rate.
- Elevated immunoglobulin levels.
- Positive rheumatoid factor.
- Low complement levels.
- *Note:* when doing lab, remember to screen for hepatitis.

Gout

- Usually affects one joint in lower extremity.
- Joint tap is inflammatory (50,000/mm^3 neutrophils).
- Negatively birefringent uric acid crystals under polarized microscopy.
- NSAIDs for acute attack.

Allopurinol

- A xanthine oxidase inhibitor.
- Can also trigger acute gout.
- Always start with colchicine for two weeks before, then 6–12 months after adding allopurinol.
- Side effects: eosinophilia, fever, hepatitis, renal dysfunction, and erythematous, desquamative rash.

Pseudogout

- Pseudogout results from calcium pyrophosphate deposition.
- Crystals are rhomboid and weakly positively birefringent under polarized microscope.
- May overlap an acute gout attack and/or septic joint.
- Knee is most commonly affected joint.
- Often shows chondrocalcinosis on X-ray.

Ankylosing spondylitis

- Chronic inflammation of sacro-iliac joints and spine.
- Usually associated with HLA-B27.
- Lab = high sedimentation rate; negative rheumatoid factor.
- X-rays can show squaring of vertebral bodies or bamboo spine.
- May also have fatigue, fever, or iritis.

Whipple disease

- Causes palindromic rheumatism (a severe, recurrent, unpredictable arthritis, usually of 1–2 joints at a time).
- Patients have recurrent, chronic diarrhea for years.
- Constitutional symptoms are present (fever, fatigue, and lymphadenopathy).
- Caused by the intracellular bacterium *Tropheryma whipplei* (formerly *T. whippelii*)
- *Tropheryma whipplei* can also cause culture-negative endocarditis, encephalitis, and uveitis.

Diffuse hypertrophic skeletal hyperostosis (DISH)

- Patient feels stiffness in spine, but has relatively well-preserved spine motion.
- Diagnosis: X-ray shows "flowing" ossification on anterolateral aspect of four or more contiguous vertebral bodies.
- Disc height is preserved.

Psoriatic arthritis

- Nail pitting.
- X-rays can show "sausage finger" and "pencil in cup" deformity.
- DIP joint erosions.

Systemic lupus erythematosus (SLE)

- Malar rash, arthritis, and photosensitivity.
- Also: seizures, pleuritis, and pericarditis.
- Lab diagnosis: anti-Smith Ab, anticardiolipin antibodies, lupus anticoagulant, ANA, anti-nDNA Ab; complement is often low.
- May also see proteinuria, anemia, leukopenia, lymphopenia, or thrombocytopenia.

Drug-induced lupus

- Hydralazine and procainamide.
- ANA often positive.
- Very commonly presents with arthralgias and polyarthritis.
- Pericarditis or pleural effusion often seen.

Lupus anticoagulant testing

- Prothrombin time (PT) is normal.
- Partial thromboplastin time (PTT) prolonged.
- Clotting time prolonged.
- Diagnostic key: prolonged PTT is not corrected by adding normal plasma.

Systemic sclerosis (Scleroderma)

- Symmetrical induration of finger skin, sclerodactyly, fingertip pitting, and bibasilar pulmonary fibrosis.
- Raynaud syndrome invariably occurs.
- Cardiac conduction defects common.
- ACE-inhibitor meds are best for hypertension in these patients.
- Lab clue: anti-Scl-70.
- Also may see an elevated anticentromere antibody, especially in CREST variant.

Limited scleroderma (CREST syndrome)

- Calcinosis.
- Raynaud.
- Esophageal dysmotility.
- Sclerodactyly.
- Telangiectasias.

Raynaud phenomenon

- Vasospastic disorder.
- Episodic color changes of blanching, cyanosis, and hyperemia.
- Triggered by cold or emotional stress.
- Female predominance.
- Treat with gloves and calcium channel blockers.
- Beta blockers are contraindicated.

Reiter syndrome

- Classic triad of arthritis, nongonococcal urethritis, and conjunctivitis.
- Often associated with human leukocyte antigen (HLA)–B27.
- Associated bacteria include Shigella, Salmonella, *Streptococcus viridans*, Mycoplasma, Cyclospora, Chlamydia, and Yersinia.
- Arthritis symptoms usually occur 1–3 weeks after the initial episode of urethritis, cervicitis, or diarrhea.
- Look for asymmetric joint pain, low back pain, and radiation to buttocks.
- Fever, malaise, and myalgia are common.
- May have non-painful ulcers (in contrast to Behçet ulcers, which are *painful*).
- May cause severe arthritis of six months or more duration, either with or without sacroiliitis.
- Always rule out septic arthritis.

Behçet syndrome

- Must have three episodes of oral ulcers in a year.
- Must also have two of the following:
  - Recurrent, painful genital ulcers that scar.
  - Ophthalmic lesions (e.g., uveitis).
  - Skin lesions (e.g., erythema nodosum).
  - Pathergy (papular skin reaction appearing 48 hours after skin prick with sterile needle).
- Autoimmune vasculitis causes thrombosis, aneurysm rupture, CNS involvement, and blindness.
- Average age of onset: 25 years of age.
- Arthropathy often involves the knee.
- Gastrointestinal involvement is common (colitis).
- May have spondylitis/sacroiliitis.

Polymyalgia rheumatica

- Occurs in patients 50 years of age or older.
- Diagnosis requires neck pain, bilateral shoulder pain, and pelvic girdle pain along with morning stiffness.
- Very responsive to low dose steroids.
- May also have constitutional symptoms (fever, weight loss, night sweats).
- Lab shows elevated sedimentation rate.

Inflammatory myopathies

- Polymyositis and dermatomyositis give proximal muscle weakness.
- Treat with steroids until CPK improves.
- Typical patient has difficulty walking up stairs.
- Dysphagia (remember that the first one-third of the esophagus is skeletal muscle).
- Inclusion body myositis gives proximal and distal weakness (and poor response to steroids).
- Dermatomyositis has a heliotrope rash and a very high risk of malignancy.

Side effects of chronic steroids

- Glucose intolerance.
- Osteoporosis.
- Avascular necrosis (diagnose with MRI).
- Weight gain and central obesity.
- Cataracts.
- Insomnia.

Osteoporosis risk factors

- Slender build.
- Caucasian or Asian race.
- Smoking.
- First-degree relative.
- Alcoholism.
- Early menopause or amenorrhea.
- Poor diet or low calcium intake.

Bone density testing

- T-score compares patient's bone mineral density to that of a healthy young adult.
- WHO criteria:
  - T-score within 1 standard deviation (SD) or better is normal.
  - T-score of −1 to −2.5 SD is defined as osteopenia.
  - T-score less than −2.5 SD is defined as osteoporosis.
  - T-score of less than −2.5 SD with fracture is defined as severe osteoporosis.

Osteomalacia

- Failure of bone mineralization.
- Lab may show decreased serum calcium, decreased phosphate, and increased alkaline phosphate.
- Pseudofractures = focal, demineralized osteoid zones.

Paget disease

- A disease of disordered bone remodeling.
- Clinical: abnormal fractures or bone pain.
- Lab may show elevated serum alkaline phosphate, but normal calcium.
- Use bone scan for diagnosis.
- Risk for malignant transformation.
- Treat with calcitonin and bisphosphonates.

Osgood-Schlatter disease

- Characterized by pain at tibial tuberosity, occasionally related to exercise or trauma.
- Male predominance.
- Usually affects people age 18 and under.
- X-rays may show calcification or irregular ossification at tendon insertion.
- Usually remits spontaneously.
- NSAID can help with symptoms.

Auto-antibody associations

- Anti-dsDNA: sensitive and specific for SLE.
- Anti-Sm (Smith): specific for SLE.

- Anticentromere: CREST syndrome.
- Anti-Scl-70: systemic sclerosis.
- Anti-SSA (Anti-Ro) and Anti–SSB (Anti-La): Sjögren syndrome (dry eyes and dry mouth with increased risk of lymphoma).
- Anti-RNP: mixed connective tissue disease (mixed signs and symptoms from several rheumatologic diseases).
- Antihistone: drug-induced SLE (e.g., from procainamide or hydralizine).

Fibromyalgia

- A diagnosis of exclusion.
- Cause is unknown.
- Most patients are female.
- Symptoms wax and wane, and change by the day.
- Pain is constant, bilateral, above and below the waist, and has lasted more than three consecutive months.
- Antidepressants and mild, non-opioid analgesics may help.
- Important to empathize with patient.

Eosinophilic fasciitis

- Clinical: scleroderma-like skin changes, but often spares the hands.
- Raynaud is not present.
- Skin becomes thickened and indurated, especially on proximal forearms and upper legs; distal portions of extremities are spared.
- Patients have peripheral eosinophilia with increased sedimentation rate.
- Biopsy shows eosinophilic infiltrate.

Eosinophilia myalgia syndrome

- Defined as a blood eosinophil count greater than 1000 cells/mL, with incapacitating myalgia and no evidence of infectious or neoplastic cause.
- Past sources: vitamin supplements containing a contaminated preparation of L-tryptophan; adulterated Spanish rapeseed oil; incidence has dropped since recall of contaminated products.
- Clinical: abrupt onset of severe myalgia; muscle cramps, dyspnea, edema, fever, fatigue, and rash.
- May cause a skin thickening similar to eosinophilic fasciitis.
- Acute inflammatory symptoms last 3–6 months, with residual effects for 3–4 years.

Miscellaneous rheumatologic associations

- Ehlers-Danlos syndrome: overly stretchable skin with joint hypermobility.
- Pseudoxanthoma elasticum: recurrent gastrointestinal bleed; angioid streaks on funduscopic exam.
- Marfan syndrome: overly long arms and legs; dilated aortic root; displaced ocular lens.

Gonococcal arthritis

- A disseminated infection of *Neisseria gonorrhoeae* that manifests with arthritis.
- Patients may present either with a migratory arthritis (with diffuse rash) or with a localized, septic arthritis.
- The migratory, bacteremic presentation is associated with the classic triad of dermatitis, tenosynovitis, and migratory polyarthritis.
- The septic arthritis presentation usually affects the wrist, hand, knee, elbow, or shoulder.
- Joint tap typically shows cell count >50,000 WBC/mm^3 (mostly polymorphonuclear cells).
- Treat aggressively with intravenous antibiotics; septic joint requires repeated drainage.

Morton neuroma

- A perineural fibrosis and nerve degeneration of the common digital nerve in the foot.
- Most frequently occurs between the third and fourth metatarsal heads.
- Clinical: intermittent pain and numbness in the forefoot and corresponding toes.
- Often seen in distance runners or cyclists.
- Differentiate from stress fracture; perform MRI if diagnosis is unclear.

CHAPTER 7

Infectious Disease

Group A beta-hemolytic strep pharyngitis

- Throat swab only 50–70% sensitive.
- Throat culture is gold standard (90–100% sensitive).
- Very sensitive to penicillin.
- Penicillin for strep pharyngitis prevents rheumatic fever.

Rheumatic fever diagnostic criteria

- Major Jones criteria (need two out of five of the following, plus evidence of antecedent group A strep infection by culture or serology):
  - Carditis.
  - Polyarthritis.
  - Chorea.
  - Erythema marginatum.
  - Subcutaneous nodules.

Necrotizing fasciitis

- High mortality.
- Requires prompt antibiotic treatment and extensive debridement.
- Treat with clindamycin and penicillin.

Other strep strains

- Group B strep: "B" for baby: causes postpartum maternal and neonatal infections.

- Group D strep (strep bovis): causes endocarditis that is associated with colon cancer.

Enterococci

- Pan-resistant to cephalosporins.
- Vancomycin-resistant enterococci are a growing concern.
- Treat with ampicillin and gentamycin for endocarditis (4–6 weeks).

Streptococcus pneumoniae

- Pneumococcus: common cause of sinusitis, otitis, and pneumonia.
- Leading cause of bacterial meningitis in adults.
- For bacterial meningitis: use ceftriaxone and vancomycin while cultures pending.
- Causes fulminant infection with disseminated intravascular coagulation (DIC) in sickle cell and splenectomy patients.

Staphylococcus aureus

- Treat staph aureus endocarditis with antibiotics for 4–6 weeks.
- Catheter infection: two weeks of IV antibiotics.
- Penicillin G can be used if organism is sensitive to penicillin.
- Use vancomycin for any severe infection from methicillin-resistant staph aureus (MRSA).
- Other options for MRSA: daptomycin, linezolid (Note: linezolid is preferable for MRSA pneumonia, while daptomycin is not advisable for MRSA pneumonia).

Hemolytic uremic syndrome (HUS)

- HUS is a clinical syndrome of acute renal failure, hemolytic anemia, fever, and thrombocytopenia.
- HUS is very similar to thrombotic thrombocytopenic purpura (TTP), but has more renal involvement; in contrast, TTP has more neurological involvement. (Note: TTP is discussed in the hematology chapter.)
- Most commonly caused by a toxin produced from *Escherichia coli* serotype 0157:H7.
- *Note:* Plasmapheresis with fresh frozen plasma replacement is recommended for TTP, not HUS (even though many centers empirically treat both the same).

Pseudomonas aeruginosa

- Often seen in nosocomial and burn infections.
- Causes "hot tub" folliculitis.
- Also a cause of osteomyelitis.
- Causes malignant otitis externa in patients with diabetes mellitus.
- It is resistant to most antibiotics.
- To treat febrile, neutropenic patients, cover with ceftazidime or imipenem; may also add gentamycin if they are really sick.

Haemophilus influenzae

- *Haemophilus influenzae* is now less common in children thanks to vaccination.
- Treat with third-generation cephalosporins (e.g., cefotaxime or ceftriaxone) or second generation cephalosporins (e.g., cefuroxime).

Bordetella pertussis

- Spread by airborne respiratory droplets.
- Damages ciliated respiratory epithelium.
- May progress from upper respiratory disorder to "whooping" cough.
- Cough may persist for many weeks.
- May get conjunctival hemorrhages and facial petechiae from intense coughing.
- Treat patient, and their household or close school contacts, with 14 days of PO erythromycin.

Brucellosis

- May cause fever of unknown origin in patients in Texas, California, or Florida.
- Seen in meat or livestock handlers, or those who drink unpasteurized milk.
- Can cause chronic, caseating granulomas; lab cultures make take 4–6 weeks to grow.
- Clinical clues: fever, lymphadenopathy, sacroiliitis, epididymo-orchitis.
- Treat with doxycycline + streptomycin.

Legionella

- Causes pneumonia; often associated with contaminated water sources.
- Clinical: may see fever, dry cough, bilateral pulmonary infiltrates, and bradycardia.

- Lab clues: low sodium and phosphorus, leukocytosis, and increased LFTs.
- Treat with macrolides or fluoroquinolones.

Chlamydia psittaci

- Associated with exposure to birds, usually pets.
- Clinical: fever, headache, dry cough, and myalgia.
- Lab: may show elevated AST and hyponatremia.
- Treat with doxycycline or tetracycline.

Chlamydia trachomatis

- Sexually transmitted genitourinary infection.
- Can cause trachoma (chronic eye infection).

Miscellaneous vector associations

- Rats in New Mexico = plague.
- Squirrels or rabbits = tularemia.
- Rodents or cattle in Cape Cod or Nantucket area = babesiosis
- Cat or dog bite* = *Pasteurella multocida*
- Cat scratch* = *Bartonella henselae*
- *Note: distinguishing these two may be a trick question on the exam.

Neisseria gonorrhoeae

- On Boards, often presents as a young patient with monoarticular arthritis (e.g., knee or ankle).
- Aspirate joint for cultures.
- Must also treat for chlamydia.
- In a patient with recurrent Neisseria infections, check a CH50 level.

Neisseria meningitidis

- Clinical: fever, palpable purpura, and hypotension.
- Lab: indicates DIC.
- Start empiric treatment immediately with penicillin G.
- Start prophylaxis of contacts with Cipro or Rifampin (IM ceftriaxone is another option).

Vibrio vulnificus

- A perennial Board question.
- Typical case is a vacationer in New Orleans.
- Results from eating infected oysters, or through a superficial skin wound while bathing in warm salt water.
- Clinical scenario can be quite striking: hemorrhagic bullae, fever, and hypotension.
- Fulminant course is common in patients with cirrhosis or immuno-suppression.
- Has a high mortality from bacteremia, even with antibiotics.
- Treat with tetracycline.

Listeria

- Typical case: pregnant women who eat soft or homemade cheeses.
- Meningitis and bacteremia can occur.
- Penicillin with gentamycin is preferred; Listeria are pan-resistant to cephalosporins.

Corynebacterium diphtheriae

- Diphtheria is prevented by vaccination.
- Clinical: can cause a grey, pseudomembranous infection over respiratory tract (especially pharynx).
- The real damage is toxin-mediated: myocarditis, polyneuritis, and respiratory muscle paralysis.

Bacillus anthracis

- "Anthrax" is the Greek word for "coal."
- Named after the dark, necrotic lesion produced by cutaneous infection.
- Also known as "wool-sorter's disease."
- Gastrointestinal form is contracted from ingesting infected meat.
- Inhalation is almost invariably fatal, but symptoms take a few days to show up (clinical signs are fever, hypoxemia, hypotension, shock, subarachnoid hemorrhage).
- Adult exposure prophylaxis: 60 days of ciprofloxacin.

Bacillus cereus

- Toxin producing strains cause gastroenteritis (emetictoxin and entero-toxin forms).

- Clinical: gastroenteritis from pre-formed toxin.
- Associated with fried rice left too long at room temperature.

Bacteroides species

- These are normal mouth and colonic flora.
- Can cause foul-smelling, anaerobic abscesses.
- Are also notorious for intra-abdominal infections and tubo-ovarian abscesses.
- Also a major cause of aspiration pneumonia.
- Can cause osteomyelitis in diabetics.

Salmonella typhi

- Contracted from food or water that is contaminated with infected human stool.
- Antibiotic treatment greatly reduces morbidity and mortality. (However, antibiotic treatment of mild Salmonella gastroenteritis is not recommended.)
- Clinical: malaise, headache, high fever, weight loss, apathy, and rose spots on skin.
- Treat with fluoroquinolones or third-generation cephalosporins.

Yersinia pestis

- Causes plague.
- Reservoir: wild rodents in desert Southwest.
- Bubonic form characterized by enlarged, local lymphadenopathy (buboes).
- Pneumonic form in humans is transmitted by airborne spread (sneezing).
- Treat with streptomycin.

Botulism

- Inhibits acetylcholine release from the cholinergic motor end plate.
- Clinical: diplopia and flaccid, descending paralysis.
- Usually results from ingesting infected, home-canned food.
- Can be found in local, homemade honey.

Actinomyces israelii

- These are normal, anaerobic mouth flora.
- May cause a "lumpy jaw" following dental extraction.

- Creates a chronic, draining sinus.
- "Sulfur granules" are formed from clumps of filaments.

Pulmonary tuberculosis (TB) treatment

- "R.I.P.E." – All six-month regimens contain rifampin, isoniazid, and first two months of pyrazinamide.
- Ethambutol is most often the fourth drug (added for the first two months).
- This is also the treatment for TB in HIV-infected patients.
- In pregnant patients, leave out pyrazinamide, and instead treat with three drugs for nine months.

Latent TB treatment

- Isoniazid therapy for nine months is the preferred regimen.
- Typical Board question is a nursing home resident without clinical disease, but 13 mm diameter induration on PPD. (Here, the risk factor is nursing home residence.)

Leptospirosis

- From contact with rat and dog urine.
- Clinical: abrupt onset headache, fever, and chills.
- Conjunctival suffusion is a clue.
- Late phase may cause death from meningitis, renal failure, or liver failure.
- Penicillin G effective only if given early (e.g., the first few days after symptoms start).

Mycobacteria

- *Mycobacterium marinum:* non-healing soft tissue wounds in marine workers.
- *Mycobacterium leprae:* leprosy.
- *Mycobacterium scrofulaceum:* lymphadenitis in children.
- *Mycobacterium avium-intracellulare:* lymphadenitis and pulmonary infection, especially in AIDS.
- *Mycobacterium tuberculosis:* see pulmonary section in this chapter.

Lyme stage I

- Ixodes ticks are the vector for *Borrelia burgdorferi.*
- Erythema migrans may occur during the first month.

- Clinical: fever, lymphadenopathy, and meningismus.
- Treat with doxycycline.
- Common Board question: Prophylaxis after a tick bite is *not* recommended.

Lyme stage II

- Occurs weeks to months after stage I.
- Facial nerve palsy is a clinical clue.
- May cause meningitis, encephalitis, or peripheral neuropathy.
- Can also cause carditis and dilated cardiomyopathy.
- Treat with ceftriaxone.

Lyme stage III

- Occurs months to years after infection.
- Patients may develop arthritis (sometimes chronic); optional to treat with doxycycline.
- Rarely, can cause progressive, chronic encephalitis; option to treat with ceftriaxone.

Rickettsia pearls

- Rocky Mountain spotted fever rash starts at extremities and moves centrally.
- Rocky Mountain spotted fever is common in the mid-Atlantic States and Oklahoma (despite its name!).
- Typhus rash starts centrally and moves to extremities ("opposite" of Rocky Mountain spotted fever).
- Q-fever has no rash (and it is also very rare to have rash with ehrlichiosis).
- Q-fever (*Coxiella burnetii*) may be contracted from infected sheep placentas.

Mycoplasma pneumoniae

- A common cause of atypical pneumonia in young, otherwise healthy patients.
- Penicillins are ineffective; use macrolides instead.
- May cause hemolytic anemia from cold agglutinins.
- *Note:* Don't confuse the "cold agglutinins" seen with mono and mycoplasma with the "cryoglobulins" seen with hepatitis C, Waldenstrom, lymphoma, etc. They are completely different entities.

Coccidioidomycosis

- Causes "San Joaquin Valley fever" (usually causes a flu-like illness; classically in Bakersfield, CA); common throughout California.
- Pneumonitis common.
- May disseminate and become fulminant in Philipino, black, or pregnant patients.
- Treat non-meningeal cocci with itraconazole; use fluconazole for CNS cocci.

Histoplasmosis

- Endemic in Ohio and Mississippi River valleys.
- Risk factor: exposure to bird droppings.
- Clinical: weight loss, fever, anemia, and splenomegaly.
- May cause chronic, cavitary pulmonary disease.
- May also cause adrenal insufficiency.
- Treat with itraconazole.

Blastomycosis

- Blastomycosis forms broad-based buds in yeast form.
- Affects the lungs, skin, and vertebrae.
- Can also infect prostate, testes, and even CNS.
- Rx: itraconazole.

Sporotrichosis

- Suspect *Sporothrix schenckii* in patients with cutaneous infections ascending from inoculation site; follows path of lymphatics.
- Classic "rose-gardener's" disease.
- Treat with itraconazole.

Aspergillosis

- Microscopic: forms large, septated hyphae that branch at a 45-degree angle.
- In immunocompromised hosts, aspergillosis may invade blood vessels and metastasize.
- Neutropenic hosts are more susceptible.
- May form "fungus ball" in lung bullae (e.g., patients with chronic obstructive pulmonary disease [COPD]); this may cause hemoptysis, which in turn may require surgical resection of the fungus ball.

Mucor

- Causes severe rhinocerebral infections in diabetic or immunosuppressed patients.
- Clinical: look for black, necrotic lesions on face.
- Treat urgently with amphoteracin B and surgical debridement.

Cryptococcosis

- Causes opportunistic infection in patients with AIDS, Hodgkins, etc.
- From lungs, may disseminate to CNS.
- Treat with amphoteracin B for serious infections.
- In AIDS, use maintenance treatment with long-term fluconazole. (In this case it is impossible to eradicate it completely.)

Variant Creutzfeldt-Jakob disease

- May result from eating meat or organs contaminated with bovine spongiform encephalopathy (BSE).
- Has a very long incubation period (several years).
- Causes a neurological disease that is progressively debilitating and fatal.
- CNS pathology features: spongiosis, gliosis, and neuronal loss.
- Brain and spinal cord of cow are most dangerous to eat.

Parasitic associations

- Cysticercosis: from fecally contaminated food; causes calcified brain lesions.
- Trichinosis: from uncooked pork; causes muscle pain, eosinophilia, and periorbital edema.
- Hookworm: from walking barefoot; causes anemia.
- Schistosomiasis: from lakes and rivers; causes cirrhosis, hematuria, and bladder cancer.
- *Toxocara canis:* from eating soil contaminated with dog feces; causes visceral larva migrans.
- Pinworm: causes rectal pruritus.
- *Wuchereria bancrofti:* contracted from mosquitoes; causes lymphatic blockage (filariasis).
- *Strongyloides stercoralis:* most common in Southeast Asia and South America; disseminates in immunosuppressed patients.
- *Clonorchis sinensis:* Chinese liver fluke; from eating contaminated raw fish. May cause biliary obstruction.

Entamoeba histolytica

- Clinical: amebiasis can cause bloody diarrhea, fever, and abdominal pain.
- May also cause distant abscesses.
- Classic lesion is mass in posterior right lobe of liver.
- Treat with metronidazole.

Toxoplasma gondii

- Oocytes shed in cat feces.
- Maternal infection causes congenital defects (mental retardation and necrotizing chorioretinitis), especially if acquired in late pregnancy.
- In AIDS, causes multiple CNS masses.
- Treat with pyrimethamine and sulfadiazine.

Giardiasis

- Often seen after fishing trips or white water rafting.
- Causes acute or relapsing diarrhea.
- A common cause of bloating or flatulence.
- Treat with metronidazole.

Trypanosoma

- *Trypanosoma brucei* transmitted by tsetse fly; causes African sleeping sickness.
- *Trypanosoma cruzi* causes South American Chagas' disease; may cause CHF, arrhythmias, etc.

Leishmania donovani

- Transmitted by sand fly.
- Causes visceral leishmaniasis (also known as kala-azar).
- Clinical: gastrointestinal distress, splenomegaly, and hepatomegaly.

Cryptosporidium

- Acid-fast organism.
- Causes self-limited, water diarrhea in immunocompetent patients.
- Causes chronic diarrhea in immunocompromised patients (especially in AIDS).

Isospora belli

- Another acid-fast organism that causes diarrhea.
- In AIDS, creates a clinical picture similar to that of cryptosporidium.
- Treat with trimethoprim-sulfamethoxazole (TMP-SMZ).

Cyclospora

- Clinical: fatigue, anorexia, and watery diarrhea.
- Clues: patient traveling from Nepal or Peru.
- AIDS patients exposed to cyclospora will develop a chronic diarrhea if they are not on TMP-SMZ for prophylaxis.

Malaria

- Classically, causes spiking fevers, chills, and headache after travel abroad.
- Prophylaxis is with mefloquine 1–2 weeks before and until 4 weeks after travel (for destinations where chloroquine-resistant plasmodium is endemic, which are the majority of endemic areas).
- *Note*: avoid mefloquine in depression, seizure, beta blocker treatment, and cardiac conduction disorders (as alternatives, atovaquone-proguanil (Malarone) or doxycycline can also be taken for prophylaxis).
- Combination treatment (with multiple drugs) is now recommended by the Center for Disease Control and Prevention, due to rapid emergence of resistance from the use of monotherapy.

Nocardia asteroides

- Can cause an acute or chronic suppurative infection.
- Can cause disseminated and fulminant disease in immunocompromised hosts.
- Clinical: pulmonary lesions, often multiple abscesses.
- May metastasize to brain.
- Classic Board question: consider in an immunosuppressed patient who has new-onset masses in both brain and lungs.
- Microscopic: delicately branching gram-positive rods; weakly acid-fast bacilli.

Bacterial meningitis: clinical

- Symptoms come on more quickly than viral meningitis (usually within 24 hours).

- Clinical: headache, stiff neck, photophobia, fever, and chills.
- Neurological changes: altered sensorium, seizures, papilledema, and cranial nerve disorders.

Meningitis: cerebrospinal fluid (CSF) studies

- Tube #1: order glucose and protein.
- Tube #2: order cell count with differential.
- Tube #3: order Gram stain, bacterial culture, and tuberculosis culture + acid-fast bacilli.
- Also consider fungal cultures, VDRL, cryptococcal antigen, etc.

Meningitis: CSF results

- Bacterial: typically thousands of PMNs, but may show lymphocytosis (e.g., if it has been partially treated) or even normal cell count; may show decreased glucose and increased protein.
- Viral: typically lower cell count; mostly mononuclear cells, but may have increased PMNs early on, or may even have normal counts; may show normal glucose and mildly elevated protein.

Bacterial meningitis: initial treatment

- In otherwise healthy adults under 50: (ceftriaxone or cefotaxime) + (vancomycin) + (dexamethasone).
- Over 50, alcoholic, or immunosuppressed individuals: add ampicillin to above regimen.
- Dexamethasone has been controversial, but is becoming more routine (especially if patient is very sick, or has altered mental status).
- In adults, advisable to use dexamethasone in pneumococcal meningitis (or initially, until that is ruled out).
- Dexamethasone should be used only either before or with the first dose of antibiotics (not after antibiotics are already started); once started, continue dexamethasone for 2–4 days.
- Tailor the initial antibiotic regimen once cultures are back.

Viral meningitis

- Self-limited.
- Develops more slowly than bacterial meningitis, usually over 1–7 days.

- Can cause severe headache and nuchal rigidity, but shows negative CSF culture for bacteria.
- CSF shows predominance of mononuclear cells, i.e., lymphocytes and monocytes.

Syphilis

- Incubation time is 10–90 days (average 3 weeks).
- The classic, primary lesion is the chancre.
- Secondary lesions are small, reddish-brown and macular, on any part of the body. Patients may have annular, highly circumscribed lesions on palms and soles.
- Wet lesions are the most contagious.
- Tertiary syphilis affects heart and brain; may form rubbery "gumma" in bone, liver, or testes.
- Highest incidence of syphilis is in non-Hispanic blacks, usually age 15–40.
- Screen with VDRL or RPR (Rapid Plasma Reagin) but you may see false positive results in lupus, pregnancy, recent immunization, and co-existing viral or bacterial infection.
- Confirm a positive screening test (e.g., with fluorescent treponemal antibody-absorption test [FTA-ABS]).

Syphilis: treatment

- Primary syphilis: 2.4 million units IM of benzathine penicillin × one round.
- Secondary syphilis: 2.4 million units IM of benzathine penicillin × one round. However, if the duration is more than one year, then the patient must have three rounds of this treatment over three consecutive weeks.
- Tertiary syphilis (or neurosyphilis): penicillin IV for 10–14 days.

Jarisch-Herxheimer reaction

- A very common reaction after penicillin treatment of syphilis.
- Patients should be counseled to expect it.
- Symptoms occur during the first 24 hours after penicillin dose.
- Clinical: fever, chills, myalgia, headache, and hypotension.
- Symptoms are usually self-limited; treat with rest and antipyretics.

Poliomyelitis

- Although nearly eradicated, sporadic, wild-type polio infections still occur in developing countries.
- Polio virus is transmitted by oral-fecal route or by ingesting contaminated water.
- Virus causes destruction of anterior horn and brainstem motor neurons, causing a flaccid paralysis.
- No effective medical treatment.
- Oral, attenuated poliovirus vaccine causes rare, vaccine-induced paralytic poliomyelitis.
- Inactivated polio vaccine is safer.

Rabies

- Raccoons, bats, skunks, and foxes are the major vectors.
- Unvaccinated dogs are the major reservoir of rabies worldwide; also coyotes, wolves, and foxes.
- Uniformly fatal if treatment is not received before symptom onset.
- Treat animal bites and scratches immediately with a combination of deep soap and water scrubbing, passive immunization, and active immunization.
- No need to administer treatment if the wound was received from a healthy, unvaccinated, domestic dog or cat that is observed to be normal during quarantine for 10 days.
- Discontinue treatment if an animal's brain tissue tests negative for rabies.
- Treatment is the same whether or not the bite was from a provoked versus an unprovoked animal.

CHAPTER 8

Practice Mini-Test I

ow is a good time to take a sample, practice mini-test. It will help break up the monotony of the rote memorization you have been doing. This quiz will also help familiarize you with the format of the Board exam. Make sure to time this test, and please do not look at the answers in the Appendix until you have first completed all of the problems by yourself.

Practice Test I

20 Questions
Time limit: 20 minutes

1. A 35-year-old renal transplant patient develops cough, dyspnea, and headache over the course of 3–4 weeks; initial work up reveals multiple, confluent pulmonary lesions on CT of the chest and a large intracranial lesion on CT of the head. The most likely diagnosis is:
   a. Toxoplasmosis
   b. Nocardiosis
   c. Histoplasmosis
   d. Metastatic lung cancer

2. An 18-year-old woman presents to your clinic with a two-day history of marked swelling of her lips. The swelling does not itch. She relates that these symptoms happened once before after a dental procedure last year. This time, her eyes also feel puffy to her, and her voice is raspy. She also has a past history of recurrent intestinal obstruction about three years ago. Today she denies fever or chills.

On exam she has mild, non-tender swelling on the lips and periorbital area. During your exam, she also remembers to tell you that she had a root canal four days ago. Your next best lab test should be:

a. Serum tryptase level

b. Serum IgG level

c. Serum C4 and C1 esterase inhibitor level

d. Serum total IgE and eosinophil level

3. A 13-year-old boy collapsed after a swimming competition. The swim coach placed an automatic external defibrillator and an automatic shock was delivered. The patient then woke up and stabilized. On arrival at the emergency department, a rhythm strip was unremarkable except for a prolonged QT interval. On history, the patient states that he had an uncle and a sibling with the same symptoms. There were no other remarkable findings on exam. The most likely cause of the patient's collapse is:

a. Wolff-Parkinson-White syndrome

b. Exercise-induced asthma

c. Romano-Ward syndrome

d. Hypertrophic cardiomyopathy

4. A 52-year-old patient with known alcoholism presents to the emergency department for recurrent vomiting and weakness. Labs show a sodium of 149, potassium of 3.4, and chloride of 84. Arterial blood gas shows a pH of 7.50, pCO_2 of 26, pO_2 of 100, and a bicarbonate of 24. The most likely acid-base disturbance is:

a. Metabolic acidosis, respiratory alkalosis, and metabolic alkalosis

b. Metabolic acidosis and respiratory alkalosis

c. Metabolic acidosis, respiratory acidosis, and metabolic alkalosis

d. Metabolic acidosis and respiratory acidosis

5. A 42-year-old nurse presents with fasting hypoglycemia. Labs reveal a glucose of 28 mg/dL and a plasma insulin level of 75 (normal 5–20 uU/mL). Physical exam shows numerous small, subcutaneous hematomas on the abdomen. What diagnostic test would you order next?

a. Serum IGF-I (insulin like growth factor) level

b. Serum C-peptide level

c. Cosyntropin (ACTH stimulation) test

d. Oral glucose tolerance test

6. A 16-year-old girl is referred to you to evaluate her lack of sexual maturation. Physical exam is normal except for sexual immaturity and anosmia. On labs, serum estradiol, LH, and FSH are all well

below normal. TSH, prolactin, IGF-I, and MRI of the head are all normal. The most likely diagnosis is:

a. Polycystic ovarian syndrome
b. Prolactinoma
c. Juvenile-onset Addison disease
d. Kallmann syndrome

7. A 35-year-old man is referred to you for evaluation of iron-deficiency anemia. He states that his father died of colon cancer at age 45. As part of the workup, you order a colonoscopy, which shows more than a hundred polyps. Biopsy shows benign tubular adenomas with mild dysplasia. The best management is:

a. Reassure the patient
b. Repeat colonoscopy in 1 year
c. Repeat colonoscopy in 7 years
d. Refer for total proctocolectomy

8. A new, experimental drug trial reports that Glipiturd™ reduces serum lipid profiles. The well-controlled, randomized trial found that on average, LDL levels were reduced by 25 points, and HDL levels stayed constant. Over five years, 5% of the study population had to discontinue Glipiturd™ due to side effects. Those taking Glipiturd™ had a 10% incidence of acute myocardial infarction (MI) over 5 years, while those taking placebo had a 15% incidence of acute MI over 5 years. What is the number of patients needed to treat with Glipiturd™ for 5 years in order to prevent one additional acute MI?

a. 4
b. 5
c. 15
d. 20

9. A 21-year-old woman presents for evaluation of persistent, painless, cervical lymphadenopathy, but was otherwise completely asymptomatic. Biopsy shows Reed-Sternberg cells. Staging CT reveals lymphadenopathy in the axillary and inguinal region. Otherwise, the CT and bone marrow were negative. The best treatment now is:

a. Observation
b. Limited-field radiation of the lymphadenopathy
c. Chemotherapy with CHOP
d. Chemotherapy with ABVD

10. A 42-year-old man presents with a two-day history of intermittent confusion. He denied any headache or neck stiffness. CT of the

head and CSF fluid analysis were negative. Lab showed a decreased hemoglobin of 7.9 g/dL, with schistocytes in the peripheral smear. Platelet count was decreased at 70,000/mL. Serum creatinine was elevated at 2.2 mg/dL. The treatment of choice is:

a. Whole blood transfusion
b. Subcutaneous heparin
c. Plasmapheresis with fresh frozen plasma replacement
d. Platelet and fresh frozen plasma transfusion

11. A 45-year-old man presents as a new patient to your office with complaints of impotence, dyspnea, and arthritis in both his hands. Physical exam revealed signs of congestive heart failure (CHF), and lab work up suggests diabetes. The patient also has bronze-colored skin. You should recommend that his family members have which screening test?

a. Dexamethasone suppression test
b. Serum ferritin
c. Transferrin saturation
d. Anti-Smith antibody

12. An 81-year-old nursing home resident presents for his annual physical for his nursing home. A PPD, which is required each year for each resident, returns 16 mm of induration. He has not had a positive PPD when tested in previous years. He is asymptomatic, and his chest X-ray is negative. The best treatment now is:

a. Observation only, and repeat PPD in 12 months
b. Daily isoniazid therapy for 9 months
c. Hold therapy pending culture of induced sputum for acid-fast bacillus (AFB)
d. Begin four-drug therapy for TB, pending culture results

13. You are following a 42-year-old woman who is on four-drug therapy for TB. On month two of her combination therapy, she reports that her vision is becoming blurry. She is otherwise asymptomatic. The most likely cause is:

a. Rifampin
b. Isoniazid
c. Pyrazinamide
d. Ethambutol

14. You are consulted about an 80-year-old male patient who is six days post-op for an abdominal aortic aneurysm repair. The reason for the consult is "acute renal failure." On physical, his cardiopulmonary exam is unremarkable except for a lacy, fishnet pattern discoloration

across both legs. His pre-op creatinine level was 1.4 mg/dL, but post-op it has slowly climbed to 3.6 mg/dL. Urine output has steadily decreased, and a urinalysis is positive for trace protein eosinophils. The fractional excretion of sodium is >1.0 %. The most likely diagnosis is:
a. Atheroembolic disease
b. Nephrotic syndrome
c. Acute glomerulonephritis
d. Pre-renal azotemia

15. A 38-year-old computer programmer complains of a boring, penetrating facial pain that came on suddenly two weeks ago while chewing gum. The pain occurs in the upper jaw area and radiates to the upper teeth on the left side. The pain is fleeting, yet intense, and is also brought on by brushing her teeth. Physical exam, including complete rheumatologic exam and neurologic exam, is normal. The optimal treatment is:
a. Amitriptyline
b. Naproxen
c. Cyclobenzaprine
d. Carbamazepine

16. A 60-year-old man presents to you for the complaint of blood in his stool for two months. Physical exam was unremarkable except for microscopic traces of blood in the stool. A colonoscopy showed a single, bulky mass at 8 cm, but was otherwise normal. Biopsy confirmed adenocarcinoma. At laparotomy, the tumor was found to invade the fat, and three lymph nodes were found to be positive. The treatment of choice is:
a. 5-FU and leukovorin
b. Leukovorin and radiation therapy
c. 5-FU and radiation therapy
d. 5-FU, leukovorin, and radiation therapy

17. An 18-year-old, thin, male patient presents to you for recurrent bouts of foul-smelling bronchitis with minor hemoptysis; he has also had one episode of pneumothorax. He suffers from nasal polyps and recurrent sinus infections. His younger brother also has similar symptoms. Your next best test to order is:
a. Genetic studies
b. Sweat chloride level
c. Open lung biopsy
d. Alpha-1 antitrypsin level

18. A 16-year-old female student has been suspended from school for repeated episodes of daydreaming during class. The spells last a few seconds to a few minutes each. The patient seems to recover quickly. Her teacher reports that this "unacceptable behavior" occurs more than a dozen times per class period. Neurologic exam is normal. Random urine toxicology screen is negative. The best treatment is:
    a. Amitriptyline
    b. Sertraline
    c. Caffeine
    d. Ethosuximide

19. A 40-year-old female patient is referred to your office for evaluation of obesity, thin skin, easy bruising, and weakness. The next best test to perform is:
    a. CT scan of the adrenal glands
    b. MRI scan of the pituitary
    c. Single-dose overnight dexamethasone test
    d. Random serum cortisol level

20. An 18-year-old male patient is referred to you for evaluation of dyspnea, palpitations, and dizziness. The episodes last for about 15–30 minutes. Six months ago his symptoms began occurring during vigorous exercise, but now have progressed so that he notices them while walking. His physical exam is unremarkable except for a paradoxically split second heart sound and a systolic ejection murmur that increases with Valsalva maneuver. The most likely diagnosis is:
    a. Panic disorder
    b. Benign essential hypertension
    c. Aortic stenosis
    d. Hypertrophic cardiomyopathy

STOP TEST

Hematology

Iron deficiency anemia

- Most common cause is blood loss from the gastrointestinal (GI) tract.
- Common in menstruating and pregnant patients.
- Causes a microcytic, hypochromic anemia.
- Serum iron levels are low.
- Serum ferritin levels are low.
- Serum total iron binding capacity is high.
- Most specific test for iron deficiency: soluble transferrin receptor level.

Anemia of chronic disease

- Associated with chronic disorders such rheumatoid arthritis, vasculitis, tuberculosis, etc.
- Patients have diminished iron utilization and erythropoietin levels, despite normal iron stores.
- Serum iron levels are low.
- Serum ferritin levels are normal or elevated.
- Serum total iron binding capacity is low.

Thalassemias

- Inherited disorders characterized by decreased alpha or beta chains of hemoglobin.
- Alpha thalassemia minor typically manifests as an isolated, low mean cell volume (MCV), but no anemia.

- Beta thalassemia minor may show a low MCV, with mild or no anemia, B_{12}, and folate deficiency.
- Clinical: beefy tongue, paresthesias, vibratory sense impairment.
- Peripheral smear shows increased MCV, hypersegmented neutrophils, and Howell-Jolly bodies (fragmentation of nucleus).
- Urinary methylmalonic acid level is increased.
- In alcoholics, remember to supplement both B_{12} and folate.
- Isolated folate deficiency can cause cognitive and memory defects, which might improve rapidly (within a few days) after beginning an oral supplement.

Cold agglutinin syndrome

- Characteristics: agglutination, chronic hemolytic anemia, positive Coombs test.
- Signs: acrocyanosis of ears, nose, fingers, and toes.
- Look for dusky blue fingers.
- Patients must avoid cold.
- Mycoplasma and mononucleosis are Board associations.

Glucose-6-phosphate dehydrogenase deficiency

- Sex-linked inheritance.
- Present in 12% of African Americans.
- Mediterranean variant causes hemolysis after eating uncooked fava beans.
- Breakdown leads to Heinz bodies ("bite cells").

Hereditary spherocytosis

- A deficiency of red blood cell membrane cytoskeleton components.
- Clinical: jaundice, gallstones, splenomegaly, spherocytes, and osmotic fragility.
- Treat with splenectomy in teenage years to reduce future hemolysis.

Paroxysmal nocturnal hemoglobinuria

- Caused by a defective RBC cell membrane-bound protein.
- Defect leads to increased complement-mediated lysis.
- Clinical: hemoglobinuria and iron deficiency.
- May cause arterial or venous thrombosis.
- Diagnose with flow cytometry.

Antiphospholipid syndromes

- Includes lupus anticoagulant and anticardiolipin antibody.
- Characterized by increased PTT, which does *not* correct with normal serum.
- Causes thrombotic (not bleeding) episodes.
- A cause of recurrent, spontaneous abortions.

Thrombotic thrombocytopenic purpura (TTP)

- Signs: fever, anemia, thrombocytopenia, renal failure, and neurologic signs.
- PT and PTT are normal.
- Treatment is plasmapheresis with replacement of fresh frozen plasma.
- Note: hemolytic-uremic syndrome has a similar clinical presentation, except for the fever and neurologic signs.

Sickle cell anemia

- Causes hemolytic anemia, painful vaso-occlusive crises, and micro-infarcts of many organs (e.g., heart, bones, spleen).
- Clinical: may cause bone pain, abdominal pain, etc.
- Chest syndrome (chest pain, fever, tachypnea, leukocytosis, and pulmonary infiltrates) is a medical emergency.
- Confirm diagnosis by testing homozygous hemoglobin S on electrophoresis.
- Treat acute crises with hydration, analgesia, and exchange transfusion.
- Hydroxyurea increases production of Hb F, which helps prevent sickling, but it is also carcinogenic.

Aplastic anemia

- Causes pancytopenia with high mortality.
- Definitive treatment is bone marrow transplant.
- Parvovirus B19 can cause a temporary form of aplastic anemia in patients with a predisposition to hemolysis.

Chronic lymphocytic leukemia

- Chronic lymphocytic leukemia (CLL) is diagnosed by finding greater than 5,000 mature lymphocytes per microliter.
- The CLL lymphocyte is small and has a high nuclear/cytoplasm ratio, a gray-blue cytoplasm, and a smudgy chromatin pattern.

Chronic lymphocytic leukemia: staging (simplified)

- Stage 0: lymphocytosis.
- Stage I: lymphadenopathy.
- Stage II: splenomegaly.
- Stage III: anemia.
- Stage IV: thrombocytopenia.
- Note: you need to memorize these stages!

Chronic lymphocytic leukemia: features

- It is the most common leukemia over age 60.
- Flow cytometry shows mature CD23 + B lymphocytes that aberrantly express the T-cell marker CD5.
- Richter syndrome: CLL that has transformed into diffuse large cell lymphoma (clinical: fever, massive adenopathy, splenomegaly).
- Early stage: observation only.
- Treat stage III or IV with prednisone and chlorambucil or fludarabine (see staging below).

Hairy cell leukemia

- May cause a "dry tap" on bone marrow.
- Look for "hairy" or "amoebic" cytoplasmic projections on peripheral smear.
- Cells contain tartrate-resistant acid phosphatase (positive TRAP stain).
- Infection is major cause of death.
- Associated with atypical mycobacterial infections.
- Treat with 2-chlorodeoxyadenosine.

Hodgkin disease

- Characteristic Reed-Sternberg (RS) cells have "owl's eyes" nucleoli.
- The five-year disease-specific survival for patients with stages I and II = 90%, III = 84%, and IV = 65%.
- If untreated, the five-year survival rate is only 5%.

Hodgkin disease: presentation

- Asymptomatic, painless lymphadenopathy and splenomegaly.
- Unexplained weight loss, fever, and night sweats.

- Chest pain, cough, and shortness of breath from a large mediastinal mass.
- Intermittent fever.
- Pruritus.
- Any or all of the above.

Hodgkin disease: staging

- Stage I: involvement of one lymph node area or extranodal site.
- Stage II: involvement of two or more lymph node areas on the same side of the diaphragm.
- Stage III: involvement of lymph node areas on both sides of the diaphragm.
- Stage IV: disseminated (e.g., liver, bone marrow, etc.).
- *A vs. B:* "B" classification includes the presence of one or more of the following: fever, drenching night sweats, or unexplained weight loss (weight loss of 10% or more in 6 months).

Hodgkin disease: treatment

- Stage I or IIA usually treated with low dose radiation (with or without a short course of chemotherapy).
- Stage IIIA and above usually treated with combination chemotherapy using ABVD (adriamycin, bleomycin, vinblastine, dacarbazine).
- Ongoing clinical trials are changing the preferred treatment.

Non-Hodgkin Lymphoma (NHL)

- A diverse group of lymphoproliferative disorders.
- Low-grade lymphoma (small cells, preservation of follicular architecture) is usually not curable, but has a long survival time; *observation* is reasonable.
- Diffuse *large cell* NHL is usually treated with CHOP (anthracycline chemotherapy) plus Rituxan (an anti-CD20 monoclonal antibody).

Acute nonlymphocytic leukemia

- Peripheral smear may show many immature WBC precursors ("blasts").
- Cytogenics may show t(15, 17) translocation.
- *M3 (promyelocytic) subtype:* associated with disseminated intravascular coagulation (DIC).
- Flow cytometry is most sensitive and specific test for diagnosis.

Acute lymphoblastic leukemia

- Most common in children.
- Many B-cell leukemias express CD10, the common ALL antigen (cALLa).
- Often presents as a child with bleeding, splenomegaly, and lymphadenopathy.

Chronic myelogenous leukemia

- 95% of cases have the "Philadelphia chromosome."
- Philadelphia chromosome is a t(9,22) translocation that creates a fused *bcr/abl* oncogene.
- Cases manifest with a high WBC count (>100,000) and granulocytes in all stages of maturity.
- May convert to "blast phase."
- Treat with bone marrow transplant or Gleevec (oral therapy), a tyrosinase kinase inhibitor that specifically targets the Philadelphia chromosome.

Polycythemia vera

- Malignant stem cell disorder characterized by uncontrolled red blood cell production.
- Erythropoietin levels are low.
- Clinical: thrombosis and bleeding are common.
- Patients may have signs of hyperviscosity (headache, visual disturbances, angina, claudication, etc.).
- Pruritus (especially after a hot shower) occurs from increased histamine release due to the increased numbers of basophils and mast cells.

Essential thrombocythemia

- Often diagnosed in asymptomatic patients by finding a high platelet count on routine lab.
- Symptomatic patients may have headaches, visual disturbances, or acral paresthesias.
- Treat symptomatic patients with aspirin; hydroxyurea for refractory cases.
- May progress to myelofibrosis or acute leukemia.

Agnogenic myeloid metaplasia (myelofibrosis)

- A clonal disorder due to neoplastic transformation of early hematopoietic stem cells.

- Clinical: anemia, hepatosplenomegaly, pallor, and ecchymoses.
- Extramedullary hematopoiesis can lead to GI bleed, spinal cord compression, ascites, hematuria, pericardial effusion, pleural effusion, etc.
- Peripheral blood shows teardrop-shaped red blood cells.
- Bone marrow shows fibrosis.

Von Willebrand disease

- Usually gives mucocutaneous bleeding.
- Bleeding time and PTT are prolonged.

Disseminated intravascular coagulation lab findings

- Thrombocytopenia.
- Increased PT and PTT.
- Low fibrinogen.
- Useful test to help rule it in: D-dimer (fibrinogen fragments) will be elevated.

Hemophilia

- Hemophilia A (factor VIII deficiency) and hemophilia B (factor IX deficiency).
- Characterized by increased PTT levels on lab.
- PT and bleeding time are normal.
- Clinical clue: young person with hemarthroses.
- Treat with recombinant clotting factors.

Other factor deficiencies

- Factor XIII deficiency: labs are normal, but patient has marked bleeding.
- Factor XII deficiency: causes *thromboemboli*, rather than bleeding. PT and PTT are normal.
- Factor XI deficiency: a rare, mild bleeding disorder seen in Ashkenazi Jews.

Immune thrombocytopenic purpura (ITP)

- Clinical: thrombocytopenia, easy bleeding, purpura, and petechiae.
- ITP is a clinical syndrome that is diagnosed by exclusion.

- A bone marrow aspiration and biopsy may be normal, or may show an increased number of megakaryocytes with no other abnormalities.
- Treat with steroids and immune globulin.
- Splenectomy is also an option.

Multiple myeloma

- Clinical features are bone pain, renal dysfunction, and hypercalcemia.
- Radiographs may show punched-out, lytic lesions in bone.
- Patients have an increased risk of pneumococcal infections.
- Serum M protein is usually >3g/dL (less than 3g/dL in monoclonal gammopathy of unknown significance or MGUS).
- Patients often have anemia.
- Patients may also have a decreased anion gap (M protein causes chloride retention).
- Treat with combination of melphalan and prednisone.
- Consider autologous stem cell transplant in patients under 65 years of age who have adequate renal function.
- Thalidomide and Revalmid (oral therapy) are antiangiogenetic agents that are also used first line.

Plasma cell features

- Bone marrow of multiple myeloma shows atypical or immature plasma cells in greater than 10% of bone marrow smear (less than 10% in MGUS).
- Plasma cells: have a round, eccentrically placed nucleus.
- Plasma cell cytoplasm may contain white or pink vacuoles of globulin called Russell bodies.
- Note: plasma cells in the chronic form of the disease may appear mature with virtually normal morphology.

Waldenstrom macroglobulinemia

- Gives hyperviscosity-related symptoms of headache, visual changes, etc.
- May also present with splenomegaly and anemia.
- Like Myeloma, Waldenstrom macroglobulinemia causes a monoclonal M protein spike >3g/dL on SPEP.
- However, renal disease is much more common in myeloma than in Waldenstrom.

CHAPTER 10

Oncology

Breast cancer background

- Women have a 12% lifetime risk for being diagnosed.
- Three percent of women will die from it.
- Incidence is rising, but mortality has remained stable.

Risk factors for breast cancer

- Increased age.
- Positive family history of breast cancer.
- Early menarche or late menopause.
- Age at first full-term pregnancy greater than 30 years.
- Personal history of previous breast cancer.
- Breast biopsy showing proliferative disease with atypia, ductal carcinoma in situ (DCIS), or lobular carcinoma in situ (LCIS).

Noninvasive breast cancer

- "Noninvasive" breast cancer means confined by the basement membrane.
- DCIS is far more common than LCIS.
- DCIS is often found by mammography.
- LCIS is often found on incidental, histologic exam of biopsy tissue.

Invasive breast cancer

- Infiltrating ductal carcinoma is the most commonly diagnosed breast tumor (75% of cases).

- Infiltrating lobular carcinoma is a much less common form of invasive cancer (15%).
- Miscellaneous: tubular carcinoma, mucinous (colloid) carcinoma, and medullary carcinoma all have a better prognosis than the above two types.

Breast cancer: genetics

- BRCA is a tumor-suppressor gene. BRCA mutation is rare, and causes an increased risk of breast and ovarian cancer in an autosomal dominant fashion.
- BRCA1 accounts for 45% of high-risk, familial-inherited breast cancer.
- Consider genetic testing for BRCA1 and BRCA2 in selected patients (e.g., a patient with two or more close relatives who have had premenopausal breast cancer or ovarian cancer).
- Genetic testing is also recommended for patients with bilateral cancer and early age of onset (before age 50).

Estrogen receptors (ER) and progesterone receptors (PR)

- Tamoxifen is a selective estrogen receptor modulator (SERM).
- ER-positive tumors have traditionally been treated with tamoxifen, regardless of stage or menopausal status.
- Usual tamoxifen course is 20 mg/day for 5 years.
- Raloxifene is an alternative SERM.
- However, aromatase inhibitors (Arimidex, femara) are now standard. They are generally better tolerated with less hot flashes, lower risk of thromboembolism, and less risk of endometrial cancers.

Tamoxifen notes

- Reduces risk of recurrent breast cancer.
- Increases risk of uterine cancer; remember to perform gynecologic exam at least yearly.
- Can cause hot flashes, abdominal cramps, and vaginal discharge.
- Increases risk of thromboembolism.
- Decreases the risk of cardiovascular disease.

Raloxifene notes

- Indicated for prevention and treatment of osteoporosis in postmenopausal women.
- Does not increase risk of uterine cancer.

- Can cause hot flashes and thromboembolism.
- Discontinue 72 hours before periods of prolonged immobility (perhaps even for overseas flights or prolonged driving).

Breast tumor (T) staging

- Tx—Primary tumor cannot be assessed.
- T0—No evidence of primary tumor.
- Tis—Carcinoma in situ.
- T1—Tumor <2 cm in greatest dimension.
- T2—Tumor >2 cm but <5 cm.
- T3—Tumor >5 cm.

Breast node (N) staging

- Nx—Regional lymph nodes cannot be assessed.
- N0—No regional lymph node metastases.
- N1—Metastases to ipsilateral axillary lymph nodes without fixation.
- N2—Metastases to ipsilateral axillary lymph nodes with fixation.
- N3—Metastases to ipsilateral internal mammary lymph nodes.

Metastasis (M) staging

- Mx—Cannot be assessed.
- M0—No metastases.
- M1—Distant metastases including ipsilateral supraclavicular lymph nodes.

Breast cancer: staging groups

- Stage 0—TisN0M0.
- Stage I—T1N0M0.
- Stage IIa—T0N1M0, T1N1M0, T2N0M0.
- Stage IIb—T2N1M0, T3N0M0.
- Stage IIIb—T4 any N M0, any T N3 M0.
- Stage IV—any T any N M1.

Breast cancer: treatment hints

- After nodal status, tumor size is most important prognostic factor.
- The preferred tumor size for operation is usually <5 cm, or >5 cm without nodal involvement (Stage I, IIa, IIb).

- Metastatic breast cancer has a dismal prognosis; treatment is mostly palliative, but better prognosis with use of Herceptin (monoclonal antibody against her neu receptor).

Colorectal cancer pearls

- Stage III colon cancer: treat with 5-FU based regimen.
- Stage III *rectal* cancer, in contrast, should be treated with 5-FU based regimen *and radiation.*
- Surgery is often beneficial in carefully selected patients with metastatic disease (e.g., liver and lung).

Non-small cell lung cancer

- Stage I: primary tumor >2 cm from carina; node negative.
- Stage II: primary tumor >2 cm from carina; hilar nodes positive.
- Stage IIIA: tumor is <2 cm from carina or is invading resectable structure; ipsilateral mediastinal nodes positive.
- Stage IIIB: tumor is invading unresectable structure; supraclavicular or contralateral mediastinal nodes are positive; or, cytology is positive in pleural effusion.
- Stage IV: metastatic.

Non-small cell lung cancer: treatment

- Treatment of choice is *surgery* for stages I, II, and selected IIIA patients with non-small cell lung cancer.

Small cell lung cancer: staging

- Limited stage: limited to one hemithorax and not invading supraclavicular nodes.
- All other disease (metastatic).

Small cell lung cancer: treatment

- Surgery has not been shown to improve survival.
- Limited stage is treated with irradiation and chemotherapy; median survival is 18 months.
- Extensive stage is treated with chemotherapy; median survival is nine months.

Ovarian cancer: screening

- Currently, population screening tests are inadequate and are not recommended.
- Pelvic ultrasound and CA-125 lack sensitivity, but are useful in working up suspected ovarian cancer.
- Ovarian cancer usually has no early warning signs or symptoms.
- Most patients present with advanced disease.

Testicular cancer

- The most common carcinoma in young men.
- Very curable (even metastatic disease).
- Risks factors: cryptorchid testes, Klinefelter syndrome.
- Non-seminomas usually (85% of the time) have either elevated beta-hCG or elevated alpha-fetoprotein.
- A few pure seminomas (10% of the time) have elevated beta-hCG, but *never* have elevated alpha-fetoprotein.

Testicular cancer treatment

- Surprisingly to some, the initial work-up (and treatment) is with radical orchiectomy (this is done *before* staging with chest CT, etc.).
- Early stage, non-seminoma may require no further treatment.
- Follow-up radiation is used for early-stage seminoma.
- Metastatic disease is treated with platinum-based chemotherapy.

Prostate cancer

- Screening is controversial; most men age 50–70 should have an annual, digital rectal exam and prostate specific antigen test (PSA).
- Refer for rectal ultrasound with biopsy if PSA is greater than 4.0, or if PSA rises rapidly from year to year.
- Treatment is with surgery and/or radiation + hormonal therapy.

Hepatocellular carcinoma

- The most common primary hepatic tumor.
- Lab: alpha-fetoprotein may be elevated.
- Alcohol, viral hepatitis, and other causes of cirrhosis are risk factors.
- Percutaneous ethanol injection or ablation is an option for small lesions.
- Resection is preferable to transplant.

CHAPTER 11

Endocrinology

Some general signs and symptoms of hypopituitarism

- Can cause amenorrhea or testicular atrophy from gonadotropin deficiency.
- Anorexia, pale skin, weight loss, and hyponatremia result from deficiency of adrenocorticotropic hormone (ACTH).
- Hypothyroid symptoms result from a lack of thyroid stimulating hormone (TSH).
- Weakness and obesity can result from lack of growth hormone (GH).
- Usual cause is pituitary tumor, surgery, or radiation (or congenital in children/newborns).

Growth hormone axis

- Random serum GH levels are useless.
- Low serum IGF-I (insulin like growth factor) is a clue to GH deficiency.
- Provocation test uses insulin-induced hypoglycemia to stimulate GH secretion (avoid in the elderly and in patients with cardiac ischemia).
- Alternatives include provocative tests using arginine, GHRH, levodopa, glucagon, clonidine, or propranolol.

Prolactinoma

- Serum prolactin level >200 ng/mL is seen in prolactinoma.
- Serum prolactin level <75 ng/mL is probably a stalk effect (macroadenoma).

- For a serum prolactin level between 75 and 200 ng/mL, give a trial of dopamine agonist (bromocriptine); regression of the tumor and decreased serum prolactin suggest a prolactinoma.
- Always check TSH to screen for hypothyroidism in patients with elevated prolactin level.
- Treatment is medical, with dopamine agonists; surgery is rarely used.

Hypothyroidism

- Hashimoto thyroiditis is most common cause.
- Clinical: weight gain, cold intolerance, depression, and fatigue.
- Can also cause edema and congestive heart failure (CHF).
- Screen patients with TSH.
- Treat with T_4 (levothyroxine) replacement; however, in severe hypothyroidism, make sure to rule out and treat any underlying adrenal insufficiency first.
- Treat with T_4 (levothyroxine).
- For hypothyroid patients, monitor TSH regularly during pregnancy.

Graves disease

- Caused by thyroid-stimulating immunoglobulins that stimulate TSH receptor in thyroid.
- Majority of patients have a diffuse, symmetric goiter.
- Proptosis (exophthalmos) may be present.
- Patients may have pre-tibial skin thickening.
- Thyroid bruit considered pathognomonic.
- Lab: TSH less than 0.01 mU/L.
- Free T_4 and Free T_3 are almost always elevated; often *very* elevated.
- Can be managed with antithyroid drugs, but definitive therapy is radioablation with 131I (or surgical removal of thyroid).
- Treat pregnant patients with propylthiouracil.

Subacute thyroiditis

- A self-limited condition; females affected five times more than males.
- Often follows a viral infection of the upper respiratory tract; thyroid gland is often painful.
- Postpartum thyroiditis occurs 1–6 months after giving birth; then it usually recurs in subsequent pregnancies. (Note: postpartum thyroiditis is an autoimmune thyroiditis.)

- The hyperthyroid phase is followed by a hypothyroid phase, and then usually returns to normal thyroid function.
- The hyperthyroid phase is generated by preformed thyroid hormone released into the circulation by destruction of the thyroid follicles.
- Hypothyroid phase may last two months.
- Treat with increased fluid intake and aspirin as needed.
- Treatment with supplemental T_4 is usually not indicated.

Thyroid uptake scan

- Performed with radioactive iodine (131I or 123I).
- Avoid in pregnant patients and in severe hyperthyroidism.
- Uptake is diffusely increased in Graves disease.
- Uptake is decreased in thyroiditis.
- "Cold" nodules represent minimal uptake; perform fine needle aspiration.

Acromegaly: signs

- Prominent jaw and forehead; wide nose.
- Large hands and feet.
- Macroglossia and prominent supraorbital ridges.
- Oily, sweaty, dough-like skin.
- *Note:* acromegaly is associated with increased colon polyps, hypertension and glucose intolerance; also, obstructive sleep apnea and increased risk of heart failure and death from cardiovascular disease.

Acromegaly: diagnosis

- GH is secreted in pulsatile fashion, so random serum levels are useless for diagnosis.
- IGF-I is the best screening test.
- If equivocal, do an oral glucose tolerance test (acromegalics will fail to suppress their GH to less than 1 ng/ML).

Acromegaly: treatment

- Surgical excision of tumor is the optimal treatment.
- Radiotherapy is another option.
- Medical therapy: octreotide can often help normalize GH and IGF-I levels and shrink the tumor.

- Side effects of octreotide are gallstones, glucose intolerance, GI distress, and low blood pressure.
- Patients also can often benefit from dopamine agonists.

Diabetes insipidus (DI): background

- "Insipid" means "no taste" (e.g., your urine is not "tasty" because it has low sodium).
- Clinical: polyuria and polydipsia.
- Antidiuretic hormone (ADH) normally controls water reabsorption in the renal collecting ducts.
- Diabetes insipidus results either from low ADH production or lack of renal responsiveness to it.

Diabetes insipidus: diagnosis

- Lab clue: dilute urine with a relatively high serum sodium and osmolarity.
- Absence of nocturia suggests psychogenic polydipsia.
- After a water deprivation test, DI shows plasma osmolality >295 mOSM/kg and urine osmolality <300 mOSM/kg.
- Next, inject 1 μg desmopressin: if the urine OSM increases by 50% or greater, then it is central DI.

Diabetes insipidus: treatment

- For central DI, desmopressin is the treatment of choice.
- Desmopressin (DDAVP) is a synthetic analogue of vasopressin.
- For nephrogenic DI, treat with thiazide diuretics and a low-solute diet.

Syndrome of inappropriate antidiuretic hormone secretion (SIADH): background

- Has many causes (including paraneoplastic).
- Normally, the posterior pituitary releases ADH in response to high serum osmolality.
- SIADH is characterized by hyponatremia, low serum osmolality, and inappropriately concentrated urine.

SIADH: diagnosis

- The Board question in this case is usually clear.
- If you see a urine osmolality >500, then SIADH is the most likely diagnosis.

- If you prefer to follow the strict criteria: SIADH is defined by low serum sodium (<135 mEq/L), low plasma osmolality (<280 mOsm/kg), concentrated urine (>100 mOsm/kg water), and high urine sodium (>20 mEq/L)—except during sodium restriction.
- Diagnosis also requires clinical euvolemia and normal renal, adrenal, and thyroid function.

SIADH: treatment

- Water restriction to 800–1,000 mL/day.
- Optional: demeclocycline—blocks ADH at renal collecting duct by impairing cyclic AMP. Mimics nephrogenic DI.
- Rarely, you can give a small, hypertonic saline dose for sodium <110–120 in a patient with acute neurological signs; but unfortunately this can cause central pontine myelinolysis.

Primary hyperparathyroidism

- Parathyroid hormone raises serum calcium and lowers serum phosphorus.
- Eighty-five percent of primary hyperparathyroidism results from a single adenoma; 15% have hypertrophy of all parathyroid glands.
- A small number are from malignancy.

Secondary hyperparathyroidism

- Elevated parathyroid hormone secondary to low calcium, high phosphorus, or vitamin D deficiency.
- Typically *not* accompanied by calcium elevations.

Tertiary hyperparathyroidism

- The parathyroid glands become hyperplastic from long-term stimulation.
- This prolonged stimulation to release PTH results from chronically low circulating calcium, low vitamin D, and/or high phosphorus.
- The most frequent causes are chronic renal failure, rickets, and malabsorption syndromes.

Hereditary multiple endocrine neoplasia (MEN) syndromes

- Hereditary hyperparathyroidism usually from multiple endocrine neoplasia (MEN).

- MEN 1 = hyperparathyroidism with tumors of the pituitary and pancreas.
- MEN 2A = hyperparathyroidism, medullary carcinoma of the thyroid, and pheochromocytoma.

Hyperparathyroidism: diagnosis

- Check for elevated (or high normal) parathyroid hormone (PTH) levels in the setting of a high serum calcium.
- Serum phosphate level is decreased.
- Usually, surgery is the recommended, definitive treatment for primary hyperparathyroidism.

Hypoparathyroidism

- Symptoms result from low calcium and include convulsions, paresthesias, carpopedal spasm, and apathy.
- Also a cause of prolonged QT interval.
- Diagnosis: lab shows low serum PTH in a patient with low serum calcium.
- A high PTH means vitamin D deficiency or pseudohypoparathyroidism.
- *Note:* pseudohypoparathyroidism is an insensitivity to the biological activity of PTH.

Addison disease

- Most common cause of primary adrenal failure.
- Results from an autoimmune destruction of adrenals.
- Clinically: hyponatremia, bronze skin, weakness, nausea, vomiting, diarrhea, and depression.
- Can be fatal (especially during stress) if not treated with steroid replacement.

Cosyntropin test

- Used to diagnose adrenal failure.
- Cosyntropin is a synthetic form of adrenocorticotropic hormone (ACTH).
- Positive response: increase of plasma cortisol by 7 μg/dL from baseline, or to absolute level >18 μg/dL.

- Normal response excludes Addison disease (but does not exclude new onset or partial ACTH deficiency).

ACTH–adrenocortical axis notes

- A normal plasma cortisol level does not guarantee an adequate ACTH mechanism.
- The cosyntropin test (ACTH stimulation) does not distinguish between ACTH deficiency and primary adrenal insufficiency.
- You also need to measure plasma ACTH (low = pituitary dysfunction, high = primary adrenal insufficiency).

ACTH deficiency: treatment

- Use a glucocorticoid such as hydrocortisone 10 mg Q AM and 5 mg in afternoon.
- Alternative: prednisone 5 mg/day.
- Increase dose during stress or illness.
- For combined ACTH and TSH deficiency, start glucocorticoid first, and thyroid replacement later, to avoid precipitating an acute adrenocortical crisis.

Cushing syndrome

- Any condition of excess glucocorticoids.
- Usually from exogenous glucocorticoids.
- In contrast, Cushing disease is endogenous (from an ACTH-producing pituitary adenoma).
- Clinical: look for central obesity, thin skin, easy bruising, and proximal muscle weakness. Also, ongoing weight gain, moon facies, wide purple stria, new diabetes, or hypertension.
- Best screening test is a 24-hour urinary free cortisol excretion (more sensitive).

Dexamethasone suppression test

- The low-dose, two-day dexamethasone suppression test is more specific than an overnight, single-dose test.
- The low-dose, two-day test is used to confirm or "rule in" Cushing syndrome.
- Give 0.5 mg every 6 hr × 2 days.
- *Note:* the actual dose is frequently asked on the Boards.

Evaluation of cushing syndrome

- Once Cushing syndrome is diagnosed, draw an ACTH level to determine whether it is ACTH-dependent or independent.
- A suppressed ACTH level (<5 pg/ML) means that it is ACTH independent. First reevaluate carefully for exogenous steroids, including high-dose inhaled steroids and alternative medicines. Then, order a CT scan of the adrenal glands.
- If the ACTH level is >10 pg/ML, you will need to distinguish a pituitary tumor versus ectopic production. Usually start with high-dose dexamethasone suppression test. Good suppression argues pituitary source and taken together with a clear lesion on an MRI is enough to obviate the invasive petrosals. Poor suppression together with any evidence of or high risk of malignancy would argue for chest CT as next step. If still unclear, order inferior petrosal sinus sampling with CRH provocative testing.
- *Note:* corticotrophin-releasing hormone (CRH) provocative testing stimulates the pituitary gland; measure cortisol and ACTH levels.

Primary aldosteronism

- Suspect in a patient with hypertension and hypokalemia.
- Urine potassium concentration is usually greater than 30 mEq/L.
- Measure plasma aldosterone (PA) and plasma renin activity (PRA).
- A (PA/PRA) ratio >20 suggests primary aldosteronism.
- Selective adrenal venous sampling is the best way to localize the source of the aldosterone (e.g., bilateral adrenal hyperplasia versus an adenoma).

Kallmann syndrome

- Hypogonadotropic hypogonadism and anosmia.
- Requires replacement of sex steroids to induce and maintain sexual maturation.
- Fertility can be restored with exogenous gonadotropins or gonadotropin-releasing hormone pump therapy.

Polycystic Ovarian Syndrome (PCO)

- Characterized by anovulation; presents with erratic menstruation.
- Hyperandrogenism is manifest as excess body hair in a male distribution pattern (and acne).

- Patients often show obesity and diabetes mellitus.
- Do not rely on sonography alone: 20% of PCO patients do not have polycystic ovaries, while 20% of normal women do have ovarian cysts.

Polycystic Ovarian Syndrome: treatment

- Diet and exercise cause significant improvement.
- Metformin increases ovulation by severalfold.
- Clomiphene citrate can be added to increase fertility.
- If patient does not desire pregnancy, she can treat hirsutism with oral contraceptive pills and spironolactone (warning: teratogenic!).

Hypoglycemia workup

- Hypoglycemia is formally defined by Whipple triad.
- Whipple triad: symptoms of hypoglycemia, measured glucose <50, and clinical improvement after administration of glucose.
- If insulin levels are high, measure C-peptide to see if it is endogenous (insulinoma) versus exogenous (surreptitious insulin use).
- C-peptide levels will be undetectable in surreptitious insulin injection.
- Also screen urine for sulfonureas in order to rule out surreptitious abuse.

Congenital Adrenal Hyperplasia

- Mutations in adrenal steroid biosynthesis.
- Patients may show clinical signs of cortisol deficiency, aldosterone deficiency, or both.
- Patients may also show signs of excess adrenocortical hormones, including virilization (from adrenal androgens) or hypertension (from intermediates with mineralocorticoid activity).
- A salt wasting crisis can present during infancy; it manifests as dehydration, hypotension, hyponatremia, and hyperkalemia.

Pheochromocytoma

- Clinical: paroxysmal or refractory hypertension.
- Ten percent occur outside of adrenal gland.
- Ten percent are bilateral.
- Ten percent are malignant.
- Screen with 24-hour urine for metanephrines.
- Begin treatment with phenoxybenzamine (alpha blocker) pending surgery.

Familial hypercholesterolemia

* Autosomal dominant disorder characterized by missing or very defective low-density lipoprotein receptors.
* Incidence of heterozygous (less severe) form is about 1 in 500.
* Lab: shows very high total cholesterol and low-density lipoprotein cholesterol.
* Heterozygotes show early onset coronary artery disease; may also have tendon xanthomas and recurrent Achilles tendonitis.

CHAPTER 12

Nephrology

Acute renal failure (ARF)

- Defined as a decline in glomerular filtration rate (GFR) that occurs over a period of minutes to a few days.
- Called rapidly progressive renal failure (RPRF) when occurs over a few weeks.
- Common causes are urinary obstruction or acute tubular necrosis (from sepsis, shock, or nephrotoxic drugs).
- Immunologic injury or vasculitis typically causes RPRF.

Glomerulonephritis

- Often a transient, acute inflammatory process primarily involving the glomeruli.
- Can become permanent if not treated.
- Hematuria (with or without proteinuria) occurs with very high positive predictive values.
- Characterized by an acute drop in GFR, along with salt and water retention.
- Expansion of extra-cellular fluid leads to hypertension and pulmonary congestion.
- Urinary sediment shows red blood cells (RBCs), RBC casts, and proteinuria.

Tubulointerstitial nephritis

- An inflammatory process (usually of the renal interstitium) that causes damage to renal tubules.

- Urine sediment shows RBCs and RBC casts, but lesser proteinuria than in glomerulonephritis.
- Proteinuria also has smaller molecular weight (e.g., not albumin).
- Also look for urine white blood cells (WBCs), urine eosinophils, and serum eosinophils. (Note: eosinophils have a low specificity.)

Rapidly progressive renal failure from Group A strep

- Group A beta-hemolytic strep (GABHS) can cause acute nephritis.
- Immune complexes deposit in glomerular capillary walls, causing transient inflammation.
- The GFR drops, has variable course, and then usually returns to normal within a few weeks; most patients recover well.
- Second episodes are rare.

Group A beta-hemolytic strep nephritis labs

- Proteinuria is usually less than 3 g per day.
- "Fractional excretion of sodium" (FeNa) is usually less than 1%.
- C_3 and total complement levels may be decreased.
- Pharyngeal infection associated with antistreptolysin-O.
- Skin infection: associated with anti-Dnase B.
- A convalescent ASO titer is the key to nailing the diagnosis.

Chronic kidney disease

- Formerly called "chronic renal failure."
- Characterized by destruction of the nephrons.
- Duration is longer than 3–6 months; usually several years.
- Use ultrasound to look for bilateral reduction of kidney size.
- May also have anemia, hyperphosphatemia, and hypocalcemia.

Secondary hyperparathyroidism in chronic renal failure

- Secondary hyperparathyroidism commonly develops in end stage renal disease (ESRD). Causes include:
  - Decreased renal synthesis of 1,25-dihydroxyvitamin D (treat with vitamin D analogs).
  - Hypocalcemia (treat with calcium supplementation).

- Hyperphosphatemia (treat with dietary restriction and oral phosphate binders).

Nephrotic syndrome

- Characterized by massive proteinuria (usually >4g/day on a Board question).
- Syndrome also includes hypoalbuminemia, elevated lipids, and edema.
- *Minimal change disease* (MCD) is most common cause in children.
- Minimal change disease *should* be treated with steroids!
- *Note:* Nephrotic range proteinuria does not always mean nephrotic syndrome.

Differential of "pre-renal" acute renal failure

- Hypovolemia.
- Low cardiac output.
- Decreased systemic vascular resistance (e.g., sepsis).
- Impaired autoregulation of renal perfusion (e.g., from NSAIDs or ACE-inhibitors).

Differential of "intra-renal" acute renal failure

- Glomerular injury (glomerulonephritis, vasculitis, thrombotic thrombocytopenic purpura [TTP], disseminated intravascular coagulation [DIC], emolytic-uremic syndromes, systemic lupus erythematous [SLE], etc.).
- Nephritis (ischemia, toxins, allergic, infectious).
- Tubular deposition (myeloma, uric acid).
- Renal transplant rejection.
- . . . and many more!

Differential of "post-renal" acute renal failure

- Obstruction may occur from:
  - Calculi.
  - Urethral stricture.
  - Prostatic hypertrophy.
  - Malignancy.
  - Neurogenic bladder.

Note: order renal ultrasound to look for hydronephrosis (a good screening test).

Hepatorenal syndrome

- Is a diagnosis of exclusion.
- Occurs in liver failure (e.g., advanced cirrhosis).
- Characterized by intrarenal vasoconstriction and sodium retention, but patients are euvolemic.
- Paracentesis or diuretics may accelerate the symptoms.
- Often progresses to death despite optimal supportive treatment.
- Lab: urine sodium is less than 10 (undetectable).
- Two types: Type I (rapid death within days); Type II (indolent).

Contrast nephropathy

- Impairment in GFR is immediate.
- BUN and creatinine rise acutely for a few days following radiocontrast exposure.
- Usually self-limited.
- Worse in diabetes mellitus, myeloma, congestive heart failure [CHF] and renal failure patients.
- Iso-osmolar contrast, volume expansion, and acetylcysteine may help.

Light-chain deposition disease

- Manifests as renal insufficiency, proteinuria, and nephrotic syndrome.
- Fifty percent of cases are associated with multiple myeloma or lymphoproliferative disease.
- Eighty-five percent of cases have kappa light-chain deposition.
- Check serum and urine electrophoresis with immunofixation to look for monoclonal protein; order renal biopsy to confirm.
- May treat with prednisone and melphalan.
- Typical Board question: older patient with renal failure, anemia, and proteinuria; check serum protein electrophoresis (SPEP).

Poststreptococcal glomerulonephritis diagnosis

- Occurs 10 days after pharyngitis, or two weeks after skin infection (impetigo) from a nephritic strain of GABHS.
- May be mild or severe (hematuria, headache, malaise, vomiting).
- On exam, patients have hypervolemia, hypertension, and edema.
- Treat with antibiotics and supportive measures; excellent prognosis.
- Differential diagnosis = IgA nephropathy; but the time course is often the differentiating feature.

IgA nephropathy

- Also known as "Berger disease", related to Henoch-Schönlein purpura (may even be part of the same disease spectrum).
- Patients present with intermittent, gross hematuria (most common cause worldwide).
- Triggered 1–2 days after upper respiratory infection [URI], gastroenteritis, vaccination, or intense exercise.
- Often has a variable, relapsing course over years.

Goodpasture syndrome

- Antiglomerular basement membrane (anti-GBM) disease that affects lung and kidney.
- Autoantibodies attack alpha-3 chain of type IV collagen (alpha-3 chain is preferentially expressed in lung and kidney basement membrane).
- Clinical: hematuria and pulmonary hemorrhage.
- Lab: anti-GBM antibodies in serum.
- Treatment involves plasmapheresis, prednisone, and cyclophosphamide or azathioprine.

Renal amyloid

- Usually gives nephrotic-range proteinuria and decreased GFR.
- Hypertension (HTN) in 25% of cases; multiple myeloma overlaps in 15% of cases.
- May show enlarged kidneys on ultrasound.
- Most patients die within 12 months of diagnosis.
- Rectal biopsy or abdominal fat pad aspirate are easier than renal biopsy; "apple-green birefringence" is pathognomonic.

Renal artery stenosis (RAS)

- May cause up to 10% of cases of HTN.
- May cause up to 20% of advanced renal disease in patients more than 50 years old.
- Atherosclerosis is the most common cause in adults.
- More common in whites.
- Think of RAS in a patient who develops new-onset or worsening HTN in their 50s and 60s, in patients with flash pulmonary edema, or in patients who develop ARF following administration of an ACE-inhibitor.

Renal artery stenosis: diagnosis

- Magnetic resonance angiography (MRA) and spiral CT are the first-line screening tests now. Risk stratification helps determine the right test:
  - High risk: MRA or spiral CT.
  - Medium risk: MRA, spiral CT, or Duplex ultrasound.
  - Low risk: no screening recommended.
- With CKD, look for asymmetric renal sizes, unexplained ARF, bland sediment, and flash pulmonary edema.
- *Notes:* Duplex screening is an option if expertise is available; MRA is preferred over spiral CT. Ultrasound has a low sensitivity and specificity.

Renal artery stenosis: treatment

- Treatment is based on unilateral versus bilateral disease, based on the patient's age, and based on the location of the stenosis and risk factor reduction.
- *Unilateral:* Use ACE-inhibitor or angiotensin II receptor antagonist blockers and possible percutaneous revascularization; surgical revascularization if diffuse disease.
- *Bilateral:* Can try ACE-inhibitor or angiotensin II receptor antagonist blockers, but requires careful monitoring. For younger patients (60–65) with new-onset disease, can use a percutaneous stent. Use surgery if the above fails or if aortic surgery is needed.

Polycystic kidney disease

- Autosomal dominant polycystic kidney disease (ADPKD) is one of the most common inherited diseases.
- Accounts for 10% of patients on dialysis.
- Cysts occur in the kidney and elsewhere (e.g., liver, pancreas, spleen).
- Symptoms usually begin at age 30–40.

Autosomal dominant polycystic kidney disease signs and symptoms

- Pain and hematuria are common.
- Microalbuminuria occurs in 35% of cases.
- Sixty percent to seventy percent become hypertensive before renal failure develops.
- Ultrasound is the best screening test.
- Genetic testing is highly accurate.

Autosomal dominant polycystic kidney disease: diagnostic criteria

- At least two cysts in one kidney or one cyst in each kidney in an at-risk patient younger than 30 years.
- At least two cysts in each kidney in an at-risk patient aged 30–59 years.
- At least four cysts in each kidney for an at-risk patient aged 60 years or older.
- Presence of hepatic or pancreatic cysts (supports the diagnosis).

Autosomal dominant polycystic kidney disease: treatment

- Strict blood pressure control.
- ACE-inhibitors or angiotensin II receptor antagonist blockers are best.
- For large or painful cysts, percutaneous drainage and sclerosing therapy.
- Aggressive treatment of urinary tract infections or infected renal cysts.

Alport syndrome

- Suspect in patients with hematuria and hearing defects.
- Anterior lenticonus: a slow, progressive deterioration of vision (e.g., patient has to change prescription of glasses frequently).
- Also look for signs of renal failure: hypertension, edema, and anemia.
- Treat with ACE-inhibitors if patient develops proteinuria or hypertension.

Renal Tubular Acidosis (RTA)

- Suspect RTA when you have a normal anion gap metabolic acidosis.
- Check urinary anion gap (urine sodium + urine potassium − urine chloride); normal range is between −10 and +10.
- If urinary anion gap $> +10$, then RTA is present.
- If urinary anion gap $< +10$, then look for extra-renal causes.

Acute hyperkalemia treatment

- Treat immediately for $[K^+] > 7.0$ or for EKG changes (e.g., peaked T waves).
- First line (urgent) treatment is with calcium gluconate for cardioprotective effect.

- Next consider insulin + glucose drip to rapidly shift potassium intracellularly.
- Bicarbonate can also be used to shift potassium into cells.
- Potassium binding resins remove K^+ from the body.

Renal calculi notes

- Renal tubular acidosis, sarcoidosis, and hyperparathyroidism can increase the frequency of calcium-based calculi.
- Staghorn calculi (struvite) occur with urea-producing bacteria such as *Proteus.*
- Cystine stones create hexagonal crystals in the urine.
- Treat most types of recurrent calculi with urinary alkaliniation (except calculi composed of calcium phosphate or struvite).

CHAPTER 13

Obstetrics and Gynecology

Physiologic changes in pregnancy

- Blood volume increases by 40–45%.
- Cardiac output increases by 30–50%.
- Blood pressure decreases.
- Systemic vascular resistance decreases.
- Oxygen consumption and delivery increases by 30–50%.
- Lab shows dilutional anemia and elevated white blood cell count.

Asthma in pregnancy

- Prednisone is a safe systemic corticosteroid (category B).
- Inhaled agents are preferred for long term management.
- Discontinue B_2 agonists if pulmonary edema develops.

Amniotic fluid embolism

- Amniotic fluid and debris enter maternal circulation.
- Generates an anaphylactoid reaction and/or activates complement cascade.
- Causes disseminated intravascular coagulation (DIC).
- Very high mortality; treatment is supportive.
- Treat coagulopathies (fresh frozen plasma for prolonged aPTT, cryoprecipitate for fibrinogen <100 mg/dL, and platelet transfusion for counts <20,000/mm^3.

Venous air embolism

- Occurs during surgery (e.g., cesarean section), trauma, and central venous catheter placement.
- Clinical: tachycardia, tachypnea, cyanosis, hypotension, and altered level of consciousness.
- May hear a cardiac "mill wheel" murmur: a loud, churning, machinery-like murmur heard across precordium.
- Administer 100% oxygen.
- Place patient in Trendelenburg position (head down) and rotate to left lateral decubitus position (to trap air in apex of ventricle).
- Consider hyperbaric chamber (to compress air bubbles).

Trauma in pregnancy

- Use Rh(−) blood for emergency transfusions.
- Place patient in left lateral decubitus position; elevate hips.
- Monitor fetal cardiac activity.
- Give $Rh_o(D)$ immune globulin within 72 hours.
- Can perform perimortem cesarean delivery if fetal age 24 weeks or greater; deliver within five minutes of arrest.

Preeclampsia

- Preeclampsia is defined as hypertension and proteinuria that occur after the 20th week of pregnancy.
- "Severe" preeclampsia is defined as blood pressure greater than 160/110 mm Hg, measured during bed rest, on two separate occasions at least six hours apart; also requires at least 5 g/day or more proteinuria.
- Eclampsia is the combination of preeclampsia with seizures.

Preeclampsia: clinical

- Oliguria and peripheral edema.
- Edema is from third spacing; patients are intravascularly volume contracted.
- Headache and visual disturbances common.
- Pulmonary and cerebral edema may be present.
- Right upper quadrant or epigastric abdominal pain can be prominent.
- Ten percent of preeclampsia patients have hemolysis, elevated liver enzymes, and low platelet count (HELLP syndrome).

HELLP syndrome

- Microangiopathic hemolysis.
- Bilirubin is >1.2 mg/dL.
- AST is >70 U/L.
- LDH is >600 U/L.
- Platelets <150,000.

Preeclampsia: risks

- Preeclampsia causes about 15% of cases of maternal mortality.
- African Americans are at two times greater risk.
- A first degree relative with preeclampsia increases risk factor four times.
- Young age increases risk factor three times.
- Eighty-five percent of cases are primigravida patients.
- Diabetes mellitus increases the risk by 30%.
- Chronic hypertension.

Preeclampsia: treatment

- The only definitive treatment is delivery of the fetus and placenta.
- For preterm mothers, it is usually fine to delay delivery for 48 hours to allow for steroid treatment to mature infant lungs.
- Labetalol and hydralazine are the antihypertensive agents of choice (avoid ACE-inhibitors).
- First dose of labetalol is typically 10 mg IV.
- Use magnesium sulfate for seizures or for severe preeclampsia.

Placenta previa

- "Placenta previa" literally means "afterbirth first"; placenta implants over the cervical os.
- Risk factors include previous cesarean deliveries, multiparity, advanced maternal age, and smoking.
- Suspect in any pregnant patient beyond the first trimester who presents with vaginal bleeding.
- Due to risk of severe hemorrhage, a digital examination is absolutely contraindicated until placenta previa is excluded with speculum exam and sonogram.
- Patients should be advised to maintain complete "pelvic rest," i.e., absolutely no sex and nothing whatsoever inserted into the vagina.

Placental abruption

- A premature separation of the placenta from the uterus.
- Characterized by bleeding, uterine contractions, and fetal distress.
- Most important causes are tobacco, cocaine, and abdominal trauma.
- Other risk factors are previous placental abruption, advanced maternal age, and hypertension.
- Suspect in any patient with third trimester bleeding.
- Uterine monitor shows irritability or tetanic contractions.
- Ultrasound can help confirm diagnosis.
- High risk of disseminated intravascular coagulation (DIC).

Uterine rupture

- Presenting symptoms are often nonspecific; need high index of suspicion.
- Minutes count; fetal morbidity occurs within 10–30 minutes.
- Major risk factors include multiparity, neglected labor, breech extraction, and uterine instrumentation.
- Increased risk from oxytocin if previous cesarean surgery.

Thromboembolic disease in pregnancy

- Warfarin is absolutely contraindicated in first trimester, and relatively contraindicated in second and third trimesters.
- Use unfractionated heparin or low molecular weight heparin.
- Stop unfractionated heparin six hours before delivery; stop low molecular weight heparin 24 hours before delivery; resume either within 6–24 hours after delivery.
- Treat until six weeks postpartum (at least three months total).
- Risk of spinal/epidural hematoma when using epidural anesthesia in patients on low molecular weight heparin.
- If using low molecular weight heparin, switch to unfractionated heparin at 36 weeks' gestation; okay to resume low molecular weight heparin postpartum.

Acute fatty liver of pregnancy

- Clinical: vomiting, abdominal pain, jaundice, polydipsia, polyuria, fatigue, headache, and altered mental status.
- Lab: hypoglycemia, DIC, elevated ALT, and elevated ammonia.
- Fulminant course.
- Treatment is termination of pregnancy.

Cervical cancer screening

- Risk is increased with early age of menarche, early age of first intercourse, and increased number of sexual partners, among other risk factors.
- Human papillomavirus is a strong contributor to risk and progression.
- Board question: For an abnormal pap smear, usually your next best step is to refer the patient to a gynecologist for colposcopy with directed biopsy.
- For a finding of ASCUS (atypical squamous cells of undetermined significance) in a compliant, pre-menopausal patient, you should simply repeat the pap every four months for the next year, and then every six months for the following year.
- If repeat pap again shows ASCUS, then send for colposcopy and directed biopsy.
- Human papillomavirus testing can also provide reassurance.

Trichomonas vaginalis

- Flagellated organism that causes sexually transmitted disease.
- Creates foul-smelling, thin, frothy vaginal discharge.
- Cervix and vagina are red from irritation.
- Treat with metronidazole.

Bacterial vaginosis

- Thin, milky-white vaginal discharge without local irritation.
- Characterized by clue cells on microscopy.
- Whiff test: generates a fishy odor when mixed with KOH.
- Treat with metronidazole or clindamycin (either oral or gel).

CHAPTER 14

Allergy and Immunology

Allergy skin testing

- Prick (immediate) skin testing is used to test for respiratory allergies (type I hypersensitivity reaction).
- Patch testing investigates type IV delayed hypersensitivity (e.g., contact dermatitis); results are read after 3–5 days.

Occupational asthma

- Taking a good history is the key to nailing the diagnosis.
- Latex is a common cause.
- Typical Board question: a baker who wheezes at work (e.g., triggered by flour).
- Diagnostic test to order: frequent, serial peak flow measurements before, during, and after work.
- Treatment is to avoid the trigger.

C1 esterase inhibitor deficiency

- "Hereditary angioedema."
- Lab: shows decreased functional levels of C1 esterase inhibitor (qualitative levels may be normal) and C4.
- Type 1: low level and low function of C1.
- Type 2: normal level, but low function of C1.
- Intestinal pseudo-obstruction is a common symptom.
- Skin lesions do not itch, and they may not respond to epinephrine.
- Laryngeal edema is common.

- Episodes may be precipitated by dental work or trauma.
- Acquired forms exist, with main feature being low C1q.

Insect sting allergy

- Patients with large, local reactions do *not* need follow up allergy skin testing and immunotherapy.
- In contrast, patients with a generalized reaction (risk for anaphylaxis) need follow up allergy skin testing, but delay testing until one month after the reaction.
- Serum tryptase level may be elevated for several hours after anaphylaxis.

Stevens-Johnson syndrome

- A bullous skin and mucosal reaction.
- Causes very large blisters over most of the skin, mouth, and gastrointestinal (GI) tract.
- Infection may cause mortality.
- Well known causes: penicillin, sulfas, barbiturates, and warfarin.

Toxic epidermal necrolysis

- Clinically similar to Stevens-Johnson syndrome, but worse.
- Cleavage layer is deeper (cleavage occurs at basement membrane of epidermis).
- Patients must be admitted to burn unit (they will have full thickness "burns" over most of the body).
- Requires skin grafting.
- Very high mortality.

Churg-Strauss syndrome

- Characterized by asthma and peripheral eosinophilia.
- Role of leukotriene antagonists not known.
- Clinical: allergic rhinitis, asthma, and nasal polyposis.
- p-ANCA often positive (has some clinical overlap with polyarteritis nodosa).
- Associated with coronary vasculitis.

Systemic mastocytosis

- A clonal disorder of mast cells and mast cell precursors.
- Characterized by dense infiltration by mast cells into extracutaneous organs.

- Clinical: anemia, GI symptoms, pruritus, flushing, hepatosplenomegaly, and lymphadenopathy.

Serum sickness

- Type III hypersensitivity reaction with immune complex disease.
- Often triggered by drugs (e.g., penicillin, sulfa, aspirin).
- Arthralgia, fever, lymphadenopathy, and urticaria occur 7–10 days after exposure.

Common variable immunodeficiency

- Clinical: recurrent, pyogenic infections + hypogammaglobulinemia.
- Fifty percent have associated GI disturbances (chronic diarrhea, malabsorption).
- Pancytopenia may occur.
- Treat with IV gamma globulin.

Immunology pearls

- Recurrent neisseria infections: think of complement deficiency.
- Recurrent skin abscesses: think of neutrophil dysfunction.
- Pyogenic infections + GI problems: think of common variable immunodeficiency (lab shows decreased IgG).
- Recurrent angioedema after dental procedures: think C1 esterase inhibitor deficiency.

Hypereosinophilia syndrome

- Idiopathic disorder.
- Women affected more than men; most common from age 30 to 60.
- Symptoms: cough, fatigue, rash, and dyspnea.
- Diagnose with serum eosinophils greater than $1,500/\mu L$ for six months or more, with signs of organ involvement and no other causes.
- Restrictive cardiomyopathy is an important complication; treat with corticosteroids.
- New therapy is anti-IL5.

CHAPTER 15

Practice Mini-Test II

L et's break up the monotony again. This short quiz will help you to see if you have absorbed the material.

Practice Test II

20 Questions
Time limit: 20 minutes

1. A 52-year-old male nonsmoker with a long history of asthma complains that for the last two months he has been bothered by a persistent cough productive of brown sputum plugs. Physical exam is unremarkable, but lab exam is positive for eosinophilia and elevated serum IgE levels. You prescribe which of the following:
   a. An oral steroid
   b. An inhaled steroid
   c. An oral leukotriene receptor antagonist
   d. Inhaled ipratroprium bromide

2. Which of the following antihypertensives has been proven to decrease peri-operative cardiac events:
   a. Captopril
   b. Labetalol
   c. Nifedipine
   d. Verapamil

3. A 24-year-old female patient questions you about a five-year history of intermittent rash on her tongue. She has not noticed rashes anywhere else on her body. Examination of the tongue shows scattered

areas of erythema and flattened papillae surrounded by serpiginous, white borders. You recommend the following:

a. Diflucan 200 mg per day for 14 days
b. Nystatin gargle, 5x/day for one month
c. ENT referral for biopsy
d. Reassurance

4. A 60-year-old white female presents with a six-month history of weight loss and fatigue. Physical exam is remarkable for a smooth, beefy, red tongue and an unsteady gait. On peripheral blood smear you would expect to see:

a. Plasma cells
b. Marked lymphocytosis
c. Hypersegmented neutrophils
d. Smudge cells

5. A 17-year-old female presents to your clinic with a one week history of sore throat, increasing cough, fever, fatigue, malaise, and dark sputum. Chest x-ray shows an infiltrate in the left lower lobe. Your next step is to order:

a. Sputum gram stain
b. CBC to screen for elevated WBC count
c. Erythrocyte sedimentation rate
d. Treatment with oral azithromycin

6. A 40-year-old patient whom you have followed after her kidney transplant now presents with progressive vision loss. On retinal exam, you notice large areas of thick white infiltrate are accompanied by retinal hemorrhage, with a distribution along retinal vessels. The best treatment would be:

a. Laser photocoagulation therapy
b. Acyclovir
c. Pyrimethamine with sulfadiazine
d. Gancylovir

7. A 27-year-old dental hygienist complains of a recurrent, vesicular lesion on her index finger. The most likely diagnosis is:

a. Felon
b. Herpes simplex
c. Paronychia
d. Psoriasis

8. On a routine, annual physical exam, a 78-year-old nursing home patient presents with a 16 mm induration on her PPD skin test. She is otherwise asymptomatic and has a normal physical exam. You recommend:

   a. Induced sputum for AFB and culture
   b. Oral therapy with INH
   c. Repeat PPD in 12 months
   d. Reassurance only

 9. An 82-year-old patient calls to inform you that there has been a flu
    outbreak at the nursing home where he resides. He states that the
    nursing home had administered the influenza vaccine to all
    residents one week ago. You recommend:
    a. Oral bactrim
    b. Oral zithromax
    c. Oral rimantidine
    d. Repeat influenza vaccine (booster dose)

10. A 35-year-old, male Hispanic patient presents with headache and a
    vague history of possible seizure. The symptoms started after he
    took a construction job that serves homemade *chorizo* for lunch each
    day. You suspect neurocysticercosis as part of your differential diag-
    nosis. The best way to confirm neurocysticercosis is with:
    a. CT or MRI of the brain showing cystic lesions and the *Taenia
    solium* scolex
    b. Serum anticysticercal antibodies demonstrated by immunoblot
    assay
    c. Positive findings from CSF enzyme-linked immunosorbent
    assay for detection of anticysticercal antibodies
    d. Documented, independently observed seizure activity on two or
    more occasions

11. You are on call at the hospital this weekend. During the night, a
    nurse calls you to report new onset seizures in a 34-year-old female.
    The patient had been admitted for febrile neutropenia three days
    ago. The most likely cause of the seizures is:
    a. Ceftazidime
    b. Imipenem
    c. Rocephin
    d. Levaquin

12. A 22-year-old female preschool teacher presents to your office with
    a one week history of sudden onset, severe polyarthritis. The arthri-
    tis is symmetric and affects the small joints of her hands and feet.
    The most likely cause is:
    a. CMV
    b. Infectious mononucleosis
    c. Sarcoidosis
    d. Parvovirus B19

13. You are seeing a 42-year-old female who has recently returned from a trip to Panama. Since her return she has noted several weeks of anorexia, abdominal pain, diarrhea, and low grade fever. She appears stable. Exam is significant for mild hepatomegaly and diffuse abdominal tenderness. You strongly suspect *E. histolytica* colitis and order stool smear and antigen along with a liver ultrasound. Pending results, you recommend:
    a. Metronidazole and iodoquinol
    b. Mebendazole and bactrim
    c. Mebendazole and levaquin
    d. Observation only

14. You are following a 62-year-old female for outpatient treatment of *C. difficile* colitis. After completing a two-week course of oral metronidazole, the patient relapses and has recurrent diarrhea. You now recommend:
    a. Repeat treatment with metronidazole
    b. Mebendazole
    c. Rifampin
    d. Vancomycin

15. You are considering electrical cardioversion of a patient with recent-onset atrial fibrillation. The duration of the atrial fibrillation is unknown. Before attempting cardioversion, you first recommend:
    a. Transesophageal echocardiogram
    b. Warfarin pre-treatment for 24 hours
    c. Warfarin pre-treatment for 72 hours
    d. No further recommendations; proceed with cardioversion

16. A 12-year-old, otherwise healthy girl was mauled when she tried to pet her neighbor's dog. In addition to numerous superficial scratches, she has a bite on her hand. Your recommended antibiotic is:
    a. Levofloxacin
    b. Sulfamethoxasole-trimethoprim
    c. Amoxicillin-clavulonate
    d. Clindamycin

17. A 44-year-old female is admitted to the hospital with fever and altered mental status and initial CSF results suggestive of bacterial meningitis. Pending further results, you recommend empiric antibiotic treatment with:
    a. Ceftriaxone
    b. Vancomycin

    c. Ceftriaxone and vancomycin
    d. Levofloxacin and gentamicin

18. You are asked to consult on a patient in the emergency room who is being admitted for antibiotic treatment of pyelonephritis. She is febrile and hypotensive. You recommend:
    a. Sulfamethoxasole-trimethoprim
    b. Levofloxacin
    c. Ceftriaxone and gentamicin
    d. Ticarcillin-clavulonate

19. You are following a pregnant patient who had routine screening lab for primary syphilis. Labs showed the following results: RPR positive, MHA-TP negative. You now recommend:
    a. Repeat RPR in 2–3 weeks
    b. Repeat MHA-TP in 2–3 weeks
    c. Repeat both RPR and MHA-TP in 2–3 weeks
    d. Initiate antibiotic treatment

20. A 25-year-old female presents to your office with a two-week history of yellow vaginal discharge. KOH prep of a vaginal swab creates a "fishy" odor. A wet prep shows ovoid-shaped parasites with ameboid mobility. You recommend treatment with:
    a. Levofloxacin
    b. Metronidazole
    c. Bactrim
    d. Penicillin

STOP TEST

CHAPTER 16

Ophthalmology

Cytomegalovirus (CMV) retinitis

- Seen in immunocompromised hosts (AIDS, chemotherapy).
- "Ketchup and cheese" appearance from hemorrhage and necrosis.
- Incidence of blindness is decreasing with aggressive antiretroviral therapy.
- Treat with ganciclovir, foscarnate, and extended release surgical implants.

Hypertensive retinopathy

- On fundoscopic exam, the initial response to systemic blood pressure elevation is retinal vasoconstriction and arteriolar narrowing.
- Late effects are thickening of the blood vessel wall and hyaline degeneration.
- If chronic, opacification of normally transparent vessel walls produces the appearance of arteriovenous nicking at junctions of arteries and veins.
- More severe changes will lead to microaneurysms, hemorrhages, hard exudates, cotton-wool spots (infarcts of the nerve fiber layer), or optic nerve head swelling.

Central retinal artery occlusion

- Acute, persistent, painless loss of vision.
- Patients may reveal a history of amaurosis fugax (transient loss of vision).
- Ocular exam may show a cherry-red spot or ground-glass retina.

- Treat with immediate reduction of intraocular pressure, (e.g., ocular message, paracentesis, acetazolamide).
- Need to distinguish diagnosis from temporal arteritis.

Central retinal vein occlusion

- Presents with variable visual loss.
- Can cause painful blind eye (neovascular glaucoma), photophobia, redness of the eye, and lacrimation.
- Fundus may show retinal hemorrhages, cotton-wool spots, macular edema, optic disc edema, and dilated, tortuous retinal veins.
- Treatment with intravitreal steroids or anti-VEGF (anti-vascular endothelial growth factor) agents may restore vision.

Anterior ischemic optic neuropathy

- Most common cause of acute optic neuropathy in older age groups.
- Characterized by visual loss (usually painless) with a pallid, swollen optic disc.
- May show flame hemorrhages or cotton-wool exudates.
- Visual loss is usually sudden and permanent.
- If associated with temporal arteritis, treat with prednisone.
- Aspirin therapy may prevent second eye involvement.

Uveitis

- Inflammation caused by an immune reaction in one or all parts of the uveal tract.
- Uveal tract = the iris, ciliary body, and choroid.
- Acute form: symptoms = unilateral, painful red eye, blurred vision, photophobia, and tearing.
- Physical exam shows conjunctival injection, which intensifies as it approaches the limbus (opposite pattern to conjunctivitis).
- Retinal exam may show weak, bleeding vessels and white scar tissue.
- Treat with anti-inflammatories (prednisone, NSAIDS) and cyclo-plegics (agents that paralyze the ciliary muscles).
- Systemic work-up may reveal specific etiology and dictate more specific therapy.

Optic neuritis

- A demyelinating inflammation of the optic nerve.
- Presents with decreased vision in one or both eyes; pupillary light reaction is decreased in affected eye.

- Onset usually age 20–45.
- Highly related to multiple sclerosis (MS); in the majority of patients, optic neuritis will eventually be diagnosed with MS.
- MRI is helpful in predicting MS risk and the need for IV steroid therapy.

Diabetic proliferative retinopathy

- Hallmark is neovascularization of the optic disc or retina.
- May show pre-retinal or vitreous hemorrhage.
- Can cause retinal detachment.
- May cause macular edema due to retinal traction.
- Treatment: refer for immediate laser photocoagulation.

Acute angle-closure glaucoma

- An ocular emergency; requires immediate referral to an ophthalmologist.
- Patients may have a history of intermittent, blurred vision and/or halos.
- Clinical: eye pain, nausea/vomiting, conjunctival injection; intra-ocular pressure is greater than 21 mm Hg.
- Pupil may be partially dilated and nonreactive.
- Treat with acetazolamide, topical beta-blocker, and topical steroid.

Retinal detachment

- Clinical: patient complains of streaks or flashes of light, showers of black dots, visual field blockage, or a "shade coming down."
- Requires immediate referral to prevent progression to total retinal detachment with blindness.
- Treat with laser or more extensive surgery, depending on severity.

CHAPTER 17

Dermatology

Bullous diseases

- "Bullous pemphigoid" is relatively benign; causes tense bullae at the subepidermal layer. Primarily affects the elderly.
- "Pemphigus vulgaris" is more serious; bullae are flaccid, rather than tense, and occur at the intraepidermal layer. Higher incidence in Ashkenazi Jews.

Dermatitis herpetiformis

- Autoimmune, blistering disorder associated with celiac sprue.
- Clinical: pruritic, recurrent vesicles and papules affecting extensor surfaces.
- Caused by IgA deposition in skin.
- Treat with dapsone and gluten-free diet.

Porphyria cutanea tarda

- The most common porphyria.
- Unlike other porphyrias, does not have acute attacks (abdominal pain, respiratory failure, etc.).
- Usually presents with fragile, blistering skin on forearms or dorsum of hands.
- Serum and liver iron levels are elevated.
- Counsel patients to avoid triggers (sun exposure, ethanol, and estrogens).

Acanthosis nigricans

- Velvet-like thickening and hyperpigmentation of axillary and other flexural skin.
- Can be hereditary or associated with insulin-resistant states.
- Can occasionally, but rarely, be associated with adenocarcinoma (often gastric).

Mycosis fungoides

- The most common example of a cutaneous T-cell lymphoma.
- Sézary syndrome variant: generalized erythroderma and greater than $1000/mm^3$ atypical T lymphocytes with cerebriform nuclei on peripheral blood.
- Lesions vary from flat, scaly patches to "smudgy" plaques, to tumors. Often very pruritic.

Ehlers-Danlos syndrome

- Defective synthesis of type III collagen.
- Clinical: may see hyperextensible, fragile skin; easy bruising; and blue sclera.

Endocarditis: dermatologic signs

- Osler nodes: tender nodules on volar aspect of fingers.
- Janeway lesions: erythematous papules on palms and soles.
- "Splinter" hemorrhages in nail beds.

Rosacea

- Typically has at least three months of erythema in the center of the face.
- May also see episodic facial flushing, telangiectasias, and acne-like papules or pustules.
- Treat with acne medications, topical immunosuppressants, or laser therapy.

Erythema multiforme

- An acute, self-limited, mucocutaneous reaction with symmetrical skin eruption.
- Hallmark is the "target lesion."
- Stevens-Johnson syndrome is more severe variant.

Tinea versicolor

- Tinea versicolor, also known as pityriasis versicolor, is a very common, harmless, noncontagious yeast infection of the skin.
- Shows well-demarcated macules on trunk (leopard spots).
- Usually young adults.
- Worse in summer due to humidity.
- Treat with selenium sulfide (e.g., Selsen Blue shampoo), topical antifungal, or sometimes oral antifungal medications.

Kaposi sarcoma

- A spindle-cell tumor most often seen in advanced HIV infection.
- May involve visceral (or any) organs.
- Presents as brown, red, pink, or violaceous macules, papules, and plaques of variable size.
- Related to HHV-8 (Kaposi sarcoma-associated herpes virus).
- Aggressive antiretroviral control of HIV is key.
- *Note:* Kaposi sarcoma is occasionally but rarely seen as a non-HIV associated disease and is referred to as "classic Kaposi sarcoma."

Bacillary angiomatosis

- A vascular proliferation of *Bartonella* species, often in advanced HIV.
- Clinically, resembles Kaposi sarcoma.
- However, cutaneous lesions can be painful and rapidly progressive.
- Also, can have constitutional symptoms such as fever, chills, abdominal pain, depression, and psychosis.
- Treat with erythromycin or tetracycline for 8–12 weeks.

Molluscum contagiosum

- Cutaneous infection of "umbilicated papules"; caused by pox virus.
- Infection transmitted both by direct and by indirect contact such as wrestling, shared towels, or using the equipment at your local gym.
- Single lesions may heal spontaneously after months or years, but can be treated (e.g., liquid nitrogen) to prevent spread.
- High incidence in HIV; severity increases as CD4 count drops.
- Commonly seen in young, healthy children (e.g., preschoolers) or sexually active adults who spread it via skin to skin contact.

Geographic tongue

- A benign condition; treatment is reassurance.
- Often mistaken for thrush.
- Sharply demarcated areas of hyperkeratosis, alternating with normal epithelium—looks like a "geographic" map.

Psoriasis

- Inflamed, erythematous skin covered with white, silvery scaling.
- Most commonly appears on extensor surfaces of scalp, trunk, knees, and elbows.
- Results from genetic predisposition plus an unknown, environmental trigger.
- Flares are highly related to stress.
- Treat with a combination of therapies: topical medications, phototherapy, and systemic agents (including biologic therapies).

Seborrheic dermatitis

- Chronic, papulosquamous lesions affecting the sebum-rich areas of the face and scalp.
- Diagnosis made by distribution of rash and by history of waxing and waning course.
- Flare-ups occur with changes in humidity, stress level, or seasonal changes.
- Topical steroid treatment works, but can cause dependence and rebound effect.
- Antifungal creams (for face) and selenium sulfide shampoo (for scalp) can be helpful.

Axillary intertrigo

- An inflammatory dermatosis involving body folds.
- Typically, axillae or groin is affected.
- Skin maceration is caused by friction, heat, and moisture.

Atopic dermatitis

- Atopic dermatitis, which is sometimes called atopic eczema or hereditary eczema, is a very common, itchy, sensitive skin condition that runs in families.

- It may flare at times of stress or during the change of seasons, or it may just appear for no obvious reason. The problem frequently goes away by itself—in 40% to 50% of children—but it may return in adolescence or adulthood and possibly turn out to be a lifelong problem.
- It can first appear at any age.
- Family members will have one or more of the following symptoms: dry, sensitive skin; allergies to medications, pollen, dust, house dust mites, ragweed, dogs, or cats; or other problems such as persistent runny noses, sinusitis, sneezing attacks, or chronic itchy or irritated eyes.
- Treatment is primarily with topical steroids.

CHAPTER 18

Neurology

Transient ischemic attacks

- Temporary, focal loss of cerebral function from vascular occlusion.
- Usually lasts from 1–60 minutes; sometimes up to 24 hours.
- Signals an impending stroke in one-third of patients.
- Major cause of death is myocardial infarction (MI), not cerebrovascular accident (CVA) (so don't forget the cardiac workup).

Transient ischemic attack: initial evaluation

- Careful history and physical needed to exclude "stroke in progress."
- In acute phase, CT is better than MRI for excluding *hemorrhage* (usually done on presentation to the emergency department [ED]).
- In acute phase, MRI is better than CT for evaluating acute *ischemia* (for first 24 to 48 hours).
- Remember to exclude hemodynamically significant carotid occlusive disease.

Transient ischemic attack: medical treatment

- Aspirin is first line agent of choice.
- Role of other anti-platelet and anticoagulant medicines, either alone or in combination, is controversial.

Ischemic stroke

- Eighty percent of all strokes are ischemic.

- Use recombinant tissue-type plasminogen activator (rt-PA) treatment only in selected, acute cases (requires a dedicated stroke team or strict ED protocol).

Emboli

- Source: heart or extracranial arteries.
- Mural thrombi arise from myocardial infarction, atrial fibrillation, or cardiomyopathy.
- Valvular thrombi arise from mitral stenosis, prosthetic valves, or endocarditis.
- Embolism may be presumed based on the appearance/vascular distribution of the stroke on neuroimaging.
- Cardiac embolism is the only instance in which anticoagulation has solid evidence of benefit in reducing the risk of recurrence.
- Do not anticoagulate for endocarditis.
- Patients with a diagnosis of infective endocarditis should undergo MRI imaging to exclude mycotic aneurysm, which often requires surgical intervention.

Lacunar infarcts

- Micro-infarctions of small, terminal cerebral vasculature.
- Risk factors include chronic kidney disease, hypertension, diabetes, and smoking.
- Because of their small size, lacunar infarcts usually do not cause acute loss of cognition, speech, or motor impairment; however, some lacunar syndromes can be quite debilitating, including hemiplegia.

Thrombosis

- Arise in cerebral artery branch points.
- Most commonly at internal carotid artery.
- Arteriosclerosis and/or hypercoagulable states are significant contributors.

Stroke differential diagnosis

- Need to rule out focal seizures, infection, and brain tumors.
- With the assistance of diffusion weighted MRI, stroke can generally be identified without difficulty.

- Less common differential diagnosis includes toxins, metabolic (especially hyponatremia), subdural hematoma, positional vertigo, encephalitis, Parkinson disease, conversion disorder, and acute multiple sclerosis.

Stroke symptoms by distribution

- Knowledge of the vascular anatomy of the brain is important. For example, posterior circulation symptoms and ischemic optic neuropathy are usually not caused by carotid occlusive disease.
- *Anterior cerebral artery*—altered mental status (frontal lobe), contralateral lower extremity weakness, and gait apraxia.
- *Middle cerebral artery*—contralateral hemiparesis and gaze preference toward the side of the lesion; aphasia if lesion in dominant hemisphere. Upper extremity weakness often greater than lower extremity.
- *Posterior cerebral artery*—homonymous hemianopsia (loss of half of the field of view on the same side in both eyes), cortical blindness, and loss of memory.
- *Vertebrobasilar artery*—diplopia, vertigo, nystagmus, syncope, and nausea.

Acute ischemic stroke treatment

- Recombinant t-PA may provide benefit if given early (preferably within three hours of symptoms).
- Major side effect is significant risk of intracranial hemorrhage.
- Requires strict hospital protocol, adequate imaging, and informed consent.

Hemorrhagic stroke and primary cerebral hemorrhage

- Note: primary cerebral hemorrhage (versus hemorrhagic stroke) is far less prevalent now that systemic hypertension is more generally and aggressively treated.
- Primary cerebral hemorrhage mainly occurs in the basal ganglia, pons, and cerebellum.
- Hemorrhagic stroke is often seen following a large thrombotic or embolic stroke, especially in the distribution of the middle cerebral artery.
- Hypertension is a contributing factor most of the time.
- Treatment of acute hypertension has not been shown to be of clinical benefit.

- Treat hypertension in the presence of concomitant coronary ischemia and/or organ damage, such as acute renal failure or hypertensive retinopathy.
- Use titratable, IV medications (e.g., labetalol or nitroprusside).

Phenytoin notes

- A good first choice for focal epilepsy.
- Side effects: gum hypertrophy, hirsutism, osteoporosis, and acne.
- Rapid phenytoin or fosphenytoin infusion (for status epilepticus) requires intensive care unit monitoring.
- In epilepsy, switching from branded to generic drugs can precipitate seizures from under-medication, or clinical toxicity from overmedication. (This is due to a $+/-$ 15% in bioavailability variance allowed for generic drugs.)

Cluster headache

- Periodic headaches with a clock-like circadian regularity that typically occurs within 90 minutes of sleep onset.
- Onset in late 20s; the typical Board exam patient is a middle-aged male executive.
- Headache is intense and may come on for 2–3 months at a time, every 1–2 years.
- Pain lasts about one hour, and occurs 1–3 times a day.
- Pain is penetrating, excruciating, and maximal behind the eye.
- Cluster headaches are often associated with ipsilateral ptosis, meiosis, conjunctival injection, and rhinorrhea.
- A good history often clarifies the diagnosis.
- The first choice of drug is verapamil SR.
- The drug of second choice is lithium.

Trigeminal neuralgia

- Unilateral pain along the sensory distribution of cranial nerve V, usually radiating to maxillary (V2), mandibular (V3), or both.
- To make the diagnosis, physical examination *must* be negative, except for possible tic (spasm of facial muscle).
- The pain is intense, rapid, and paroxysmal; described as "lancinating" (or "boring") on exam.
- Provoked by tactile stimuli such as eating, swallowing, chewing, shaving, brushing teeth, flossing, or putting on makeup.

- Carbamazepine is the treatment of choice.
- Radiofrequency or chemical nerve ablation is an option.
- Some patients have an identifiable vascular impression of the affected trigeminal nerve that may be alleviated with appropriate surgery; this is diagnosed by MRI with software that can superimpose the vascular structures on cerebral parenchyma.

Temporal arteritis

- A systemic vasculitis that generally affects medium sized arteries.
- Multi-nucleated, giant cells infiltrate vessel walls of aorta and other arteries (also known as giant cell arteritis).
- Most common in women of northern European descent.
- Consider in any new-onset headache in a patient over the age of 50; it is rare under the age of 60.
- Symptoms include jaw claudication, malaise, and stiffness of the neck and shoulder girdle; fever may be present.
- Patients may have scalp tenderness.
- A history of transient, horizontal diplopia in an elderly patient should be considered secondary to temporal arteritis until proven otherwise.
- Lab studies: ESR is markedly elevated; C-reactive protein may be elevated even if ESR is not.
- The most feared complication is ischemic optic neuropathy, which almost always occurs in the fellow eye, once it has happened in the first eye.
- Blindness occurs in up to 15% of untreated patients.
- Treatment is to start prednisone 60 mg/day *immediately*, and order prompt biopsies of temporal arteries.
- Treat for 9–12 months.

Guillain-Barré syndrome

- An acute, ascending, progressive neuropathy.
- Most often occurs in the context of a post-viral or post-bacterial illness.
- Two-thirds of patients have had a respiratory or gastrointestinal (GI) infection in past 1–3 weeks.
- In children, may be caused by Campylobacter.
- Can also occur in the setting of severe trauma or burn wounds.
- Vaccinations, medications, and sexually transmitted diseases can cause it.
- Also malignancies (especially Hodgkin disease), pregnancy, or surgery patients are at risk.

- Patients who have undergone bariatric surgery with gastric bypass (Roux-en-Y) have presented with an acute Guillain-Barré syndrome that was found to be due to B1 or B6 deficiency.
- A high index of suspicion is the key to diagnosis

Guillain-Barré: presentation

- Characterized by ascending weakness, paresthesias, and hyporeflexia; usually symmetrical.
- Muscle weakness may lead to respiratory failure.
- Weakness most often peaks two weeks after onset of symptoms, but may come on suddenly and at any time during the course (usually five weeks total).
- By definition, it does not affect sensory nerves.
- Patients may have low back pain or thigh pain.
- Miller-Fisher variant (ataxia, areflexia, and ophthalmoplegia) begins with cranial nerve deficits ("opposite").

Guillain-Barré: possible signs

- *Decreased or absent reflexes.*
- Variable bradycardia or tachycardia, hypotension or hypertension, and hypothermia or hyperthermia.
- Cranial nerve palsies (and they are unilateral, unlike lower extremities).
- Dysphagia, dysarthria, or drooling.
- Lumbar puncture may not demonstrate elevated protein for up to one week.

Guillain-Barré: treatment

- Admit to intensive care unit (ICU).
- Intubate at first sign of respiratory failure; follow serial vital capacity measurements to anticipate decline in respiratory function.
- Use atropine for bradycardia.
- Give short-acting anti-hypertensive meds if needed.
- Temporary pacing for heart blocks.
- Fluid bolus for hypotensive episodes.
- Lovenox for deep venous thrombosis (DVT) prophylaxis.
- The treatment of choice remains plasmapheresis or IV immunoglobulin (IG which can shorten ICU stay and reduce the incidence of intubation.

Myasthenia gravis: background

- Acquired, autoimmune disorder characterized by weakness and excessive fatigability of skeletal muscle.
- Caused by antibodies against post-synaptic acetylcholine receptor.
- Anti-acetylcholine receptor antibodies are highly specific and have not been described in any other disorder.
- The typical patient is a young woman or an older man.
- Muscle involvement most often includes extra-ocular muscles and cranial nerves, followed by somatic musculature.
- Patients with ocular myasthenia tend to be more refractory to treatment and often have negative serology.
- Myasthenia gravis never affects sensation.
- Muscle reflexes are always intact.
- Patients typically have a circadian pattern of worsening toward the end of the day; symptoms improve with rest.

Myasthenia gravis: workup and treatment

- The differential diagnosis in patients with ocular myasthenia should include thyroid eye disease.
- Orbital symptoms must be investigated with appropriate orbital imaging.
- The myasthenic syndrome of Lambert-Eaton syndrome must be considered especially in the context of a coexistent neoplasia such as lung or breast cancer.
- Tensilon test is useful only when there is a clearly reversible neurologic sign, such as ptosis.
- Plasmapheresis is used only in the context of a myasthenic crisis.
- Initial treatment includes anti-acetylcholinesterase inhibitors such as pyridostigmine.
- Refractory patients require steroids and other immunomodulators such as azathioprine.
- Screen for thymoma with chest CT.
- Thymectomy is generally considered part of the treatment in patients who are otherwise good surgical candidates.
- Thymoma is often associated with a positive anti-skeletal muscle antibody.
- Electrophysiologic testing is useful because low-frequency repetitive stimulation demonstrates a decremental response of greater than 50% compared to baseline compound muscle action potential (CMAP) amplitude.

Amyotrophic lateral sclerosis (ALS)

- A progressive, uncurable nerve deterioration resulting in both upper and lower motor neuron signs.
- Characterized by weakness, atrophy, and fasciculation of distal limbs, small hand muscles, and tongue; moves centrally.
- Patients also have hyperreflexia, extensor plantar responses, and clonus.
- Patients may have predominantly bulbar symptoms, which often leads to dysphagia.
- Diagnostic accuracy is critical: multi-focal motor conduction block is a treatable disorder that has an identical clinical presentation to that of ALS and must be excluded with appropriate electrophysiologic studies.
- Electromyogram (EMG) is essential to the clinical diagnosis of ALS. Biopsy, while always abnormal, is nonspecific.
- In the absence of cranial nerve signs, exclude a cervical cord lesion.

Meralgia paraesthetica

- A sensation of numbness or burning along lateral side of thigh.
- Results from compression of lateral cutaneous nerve.
- May be relieved by weight loss or avoiding tight-fitting belt.
- May resolve spontaneously.

Ramsay Hunt syndrome

- Also known as herpes zoster oticus; results from zoster infection of geniculate ganglion of seventh cranial nerve (CN VII).
- The facial nerve is involved peripherally as an "innocent bystander," due to the intense inflammation of an adjacent sensory nerve.
- Symptoms are severe, intermittent otalgia; also hearing loss, vertigo, tinnitus, and/or facial palsy (high association with Bell palsy).
- May see rash or zoster vesicles in ear canal, pinna, anterior two-thirds of tongue, and soft palate.
- Treat with oral Acyclovir and corticosteroids.

Status epilepticus

- A continuous seizure lasting more than 20–30 minutes, or repetitive seizures without recovery of consciousness in between.
- Any patient who has had three new-onset seizures within a 24-hour period should also be treated as status epilepticus.

- Status epilepticus is a medical emergency since permanent neuronal injury can occur in less than 30 minutes after onset.
- The actual epileptic activity produces neuronal degeneration, especially within the hippocampus and other portions of the temporal lobe and associated structures. This damage is in addition to any anoxic or ischemic insult that may occur as a result of the motor manifestations of the seizures.
- First, establish airway and treat hypotension.
- Give thiamine and dextrose.
- Do not treat hypertension until seizure is controlled (may lead to hypotension after seizure terminates).
- First line therapies: Lorazepam IV drip and fosphenytoin.
- If status persists, give stacked doses of phenobarbital.
- While on fosphenytoin, monitor for hypotension and arrhythmias.

Neurocysticercosis

- Most common cause of epilepsy in developing world.
- Man is considered an intermediate host for the adult pork tapeworm (*Taenia solium*).
- The cysts are larvae that are viable for up to 20 years in a susceptible host.
- Following the ingestion of eggs, the larvae enter the circulation through the gastrointestinal system and are distributed primarily in muscle, brain, and subcutaneous tissue.
- The adult tapeworm is acquired from eating viable larvae.
- Cysts may cause a mass effect; also, seizures (especially when a viable cyst dies, producing an inflammatory response).
- Clinical: headache, seizures, cognitive deficits, dysarthria, and gait disturbances.
- Pre-treat patient with course of steroids before using anti-parasitic drug (to prevent inflammatory response in central nervous system [CNS]).
- If parasites are still viable, treat with course of anticysticercal drugs (albendazole, praziquantel).
- Do not use praziquantel in patients with ocular cysts (can cause blindness).

Progressive multi-focal leukoencephalopathy

- Patients have insidious onset of focal neurological symptoms that are diverse.

- Due to opportunistic infection with the JC papovavirus.
- Causes destruction of oligodendrocytes with associated demyelination, especially in the subcortical white matter.
- Clinical: headache, seizures, aphasia, hemiparesis, ataxia, cortical blindness, etc.
- Occurs in AIDS, leukemia, organ transplant, and other immunosuppressed states.
- Diagnosis is made by characteristic history and MRI findings in a patient with immunosuppression.

Ménière disease

- Patients have a highly characteristic clinical course involving paroxysms of severe, disabling vertigo with associated nausea and vomiting lasting hours.
- The symptoms are often presaged and accompanied by a high-pitched tinnitus ipsilateral to the affected vestibular apparatus.
- Tone audiometry typically demonstrates low- to mid-tone hearing loss and is a useful adjunct in the diagnosis.
- Cold-caloric stimulation will usually reveal the hypofunctioning vestibular apparatus.
- Results from an idiopathic increase in volume and pressure of the endolymph in the inner ear.
- Clinical: waxing and waning hearing loss; tinnitus; vertigo.
- Patients may report a sense of fullness in ear.
- Can become bilateral.

Idiopathic Facial Paralysis (Bell palsy)

- Characterized by paresis or paralysis of all the muscles (both upper and lower) on one side of the face.
- The symptoms often begin with pain in the mastoid region on the affected side, followed within 12–24 hours by weakness that initially may be subtle.
- Because the injury occurs distal to the junction with the chorda tympani nerve, taste on the anterior two thirds of the ipsilateral tongue is often affected.
- This abnormal taste sensation, in the appropriate clinical context, confirms a diagnosis of seventh nerve lesion distal to the middle ear and can obviate the need for neurological imaging.
- Most likely associated with reactivation of herpes simplex virus.

- Often follows an upper respiratory infection.
- Treat with oral steroids and antiviral medication.
- Eye care is important: have patients apply artificial tears as needed while awake and a lubricating ointment at bedtime.
- The eye should be covered when venturing out of doors, especially on windy days.
- Most patients have complete recovery, but a small number will have persistent weakness.

Lambert-Eaton syndrome

- A disorder of neuromuscular transmission mediated by antibodies against calcium channels in the pre-synaptic membrane.
- Most commonly associated with small cell carcinoma of the lung.
- Clinically similar to myasthenia gravis, except that weakness may actually improve with repetitive movements.
- As opposed to myasthenia gravis, muscles of the trunk, shoulder girdle, and pelvic girdle as well as more distal muscles are more commonly involved.
- Ocular muscles are usually spared.
- Patients may have autonomic dysfunction and hyporeflexia.
- Electrophysiologic testing demonstrates a marked incremental response following high-frequency stimulation.

Multiple sclerosis

- A demyelinating disease of the CNS characterized by inflammatory CNS lesions.
- Clinical picture varies across different anatomical locations (space) over months to years (time).
- Patients experience relapsing exacerbations that eventually progress to disability.
- Diagnosis is made by clinical examination in combination with MRI scanning.
- Treat acute exacerbations with high-dose corticosteroids.
- Treatment with beta interferon can reduce the number and severity of relapses.

Parkinson disease

- Movement disorder due to loss of dopamine-producing capability in the substantia nigra of the midbrain.

- Characterized by resting tremor, rigidity, retarded movement, and loss of postural reflexes.
- Many patients develop dementia as well.
- L-dopa (Levadopa/Carbidopa) is the mainstay of medical treatment.
- Most important side effect of L-dopa is involuntary movement disorders (e.g., facial-lingual dystonia, chorea, athetosis).
- A dopamine agonist should be started early in treatment to avoid dyskinesias.

Idiopathic Intracranial Hypertension (pseudotumor cerebri)

- Elevated intracranial pressure predominantly affecting obese women of childbearing age.
- Increased incidence during pregnancy.
- Most severe complication is papilledema, which can progress to optic atrophy and blindness.
- Clinical: headache, horizontal diplopia, and pulsatile tinnitus; vision loss or blurring if papilledema.
- Medical treatment: use a carbonic anhydrase inhibitor (acetazolamide) to lower intracranial pressures.
- Surgery (lumboperitoneal or ventriculoperitoneal shunting) for refractory cases.

CHAPTER 19

Psychiatry

Major depressive disorder

- Characterized by depressed mood, insomnia, decreased interest, fatigue, loss of concentration, etc.
- On the Boards, the best initial medical choice for outpatient treatment of depression is usually a selective serotonin reuptake inhibitor or SSRI (e.g., sertraline 50 mg per day).
- Elderly may present with confusion or general decline in functioning.
- Children may present with atypical symptoms such as irritability, social withdrawal, or decline in school performance.
- Always screen patient for suicidal ideation.

Selective serotonin reuptake inhibitor (SSRI) notes

- Selective serotonin reuptake inhibitors such as sertraline are usually a safe initial choice in major depression.
- They can cause a high incidence of sexual dysfunction.
- They can cause *akathisia* (motor restlessness, difficulty staying in seat).
- Selective serotonin reuptake inhibitors can cause insomnia.

Panic disorder

- Characterized by spontaneous and recurrent panic attacks.
- Persistent worrying about the attacks is a criterion for diagnosing panic disorder.
- Symptoms of a panic attack include palpitations, chest pain, sweating, and a feeling of smothering.

- Often associated with agoraphobia (fear of public situations).
- Treat with SSRIs, benzodiazepines, or tricyclics.

Anorexia nervosa

- Characterized by refusal to maintain a minimally normal body weight.
- Patients have an intense fear of gaining weight.
- Most perceive themselves as too fat (even if emaciated).
- Postmenarchal females are amenorrhoeic (missing at least three consecutive menstrual cycles).
- Bulimia nervosa subtype includes binge eating and purging.
- High mortality; admit patients with insidious decline in weight.

Obsessive-compulsive disorder

- Characterized by distressing, intrusive thoughts or repetitive actions.
- Obsessions and compulsions interfere in the individual's daily functioning.
- Selective serotonin reuptake inhibitors can be highly effective and are the mainstay of medical therapy.

Post-traumatic stress disorder

- Pathological anxiety that develops after witnessing trauma or threat to life.
- Patients persistently re-experience the event, causing distress, hyper-arousal, and avoidance.
- Symptoms occur for at least one month after trigger event.
- Treat with a combination of psychotherapy and medical management (e.g., SSRIs, beta blockers, and/or benzodiazepines).
- Selective serotonin reuptake inhibitors can be highly effective and are the mainstay of medical therapy.

Schizophrenia

- A severe, persistent, and debilitating psychiatric disorder that is not well understood.
- Characterized by disturbances in cognition, affect, and perceptions and difficulties in relationships with others.
- Hallmarks are hallucinations (especially auditory) and delusions.

- Patients may seem disconnected, with flat affect and monotone voice.
- Anti-psychotic medicines are the mainstay of treatment.

Bipolar affective disorder

- Characterized by periods of deep depression, alternating with manic episodes of an excessively elevated or irritable mood.
- Diagnosis requires a manic episode that lasts at least one week.
- During manic phase, patients may have thought disturbances, decreased need for sleep, pressured speech, increased libido, and reckless behavior such as extreme shopping sprees.
- Medical treatment includes lithium, carbamazepine and valproic acid, etc.

Psychiatric medication pearls

- Elavil (amitriptyline): tricyclics can cause orthostasis, cardiac conduction delay, and anti-cholinergic effects.
- Effexor (venlafaxine): can exacerbate hypertension.
- Serzone (nefazodone) may cause psychomotor retardation.
- Remeron (mirtazapine) can cause weight gain, orthostasis, and hyper-cholesterolemia.
- Tricyclic anti-depressants have the highest incidence of death (especially desipramine).
- Of the tricyclic anti-depressants, desipramine has the least sedation, least weight gain, least seizure risk, and least cholinergic and GI side effects.

Neuroleptic malignant syndrome

- A combination of hyperthermia, rigidity, and autonomic dysregulation occuring as a side effect of anti-psychotic medication.
- Most cases occur within the first week of starting medication.
- Patients may have diaphoresis, labile blood pressure, dyspnea, and delirium.
- Lab can show leukocytosis and elevated CPK.
- Most important intervention is to discontinue the anti-psychotic medication.
- May also treat with dopamine agonist (e.g., dantrolene, amantadine, or bromocriptine).

CHAPTER 20

Ethics

Ethical principles

- Autonomy: respect for individuals and their decision-making power.
- Beneficence: actions that are intended to benefit others.
- Non-maleficence: actions that are intended not to harm others.
- Justice: being fair in judging the consequences of an action.

Definition of competence

- Physicians determine *capacity*, but not *competence*.
- *Capacity* is the physician's clinical determination of a patient's understanding and insight for making decisions.
- *Competence* is a legal determination, made by a judge, about whether or not the patient can legally make decisions.

Informed consent

- Patient must have decision-making capacity.
- Must meet a "reasonable person standard": the consent form must have adequate information for a "reasonable" person to understand the risks and benefits well enough to make a decision.

Obtaining consent

- Physician should explain all options, then give his or her personal opinion about what is best.

- If the patient refuses the recommendation, then the patient's choice should be respected.
- Physicians have the right to withhold treatment they deem futile.

Advance directives

- An individual's treatment preference in the event that they lose decision-making capacity.
- Details what interventions they would and would not desire.
- Includes the patient's surrogate decision maker.
- Types of advance directives are living will, power of attorney, and health care proxy.

Living will

- An individual uses a living will to specify his or her wishes in the event that he or she enters an incurable, terminal condition.
- The living will may be very general or very specific.
- Does not require a lawyer to write.
- Examples of specifics include the patient's choice to have or withhold analgesia, antibiotics, hydration, feeding, ventilators, or cardiopulmonary resuscitation.

Durable power of attorney

- Grants power of attorney to a surrogate in the event of incapacity.
- Allows the surrogate to sign checks, pay bills, etc. while the individual is incapacitated.

Health care proxy

- Individual designates a surrogate to make health care decisions in the event of incapacity.
- The health care proxy has essentially the same rights to request or refuse treatment that the individual would normally have.

Death

- Death is defined as the irreversible cessation of circulatory and respiratory function, or cessation of function in the entire brain and brainstem.
- Death is a clinical diagnosis; EEG is not required for diagnosis.

Pain control and comfort care

- Terminal cancer pain is often under-treated.
- Typical Board question is a home hospice patient with terminal cancer, who is having breakthrough pain despite short-acting, oral morphine.
- Correct answer: next step is to add long-acting oral morphine, at high dose.

CHAPTER 21

HIV and AIDS

Overview of HIV/AIDS

- In high-income countries, the main treatment issues are drug resistance and managing toxic side effects.
- In developing countries, the main treatment issues are lack of basic care and unavailability of drugs.

When to initiate antiretroviral drug therapy

- First step is to determine CD4 counts and viral load (HIV-1 RNA level).
- Offer treatment to asymptomatic patients when HIV RNA level is greater than 100,000 copies/mL, or CD4 count is below 350 mm^2.
- Drug resistance among circulating HIV strains is rising rapidly.
- All patients with AIDS should have resistance testing before beginning therapy.
- Metabolic abnormalities (lipodystrophy, diabetes, dyslipidemia, lipoatrophy) are common with antiretroviral treatment.

Antiretroviral drug treatment notes

- Goal of combination therapy is to suppress plasma HIV-1 RNA titer to less than 50 copies/mL.
- The first treatment regimen has the best chance of success.
- Current most frequent first-line choices are the three drug regimens of (lamivudine + efavirenz + zidovudine) or (tenofovir + emtricitabine + efavirenz).

Prophylaxis to prevent a first episode of opportunistic disease

- Start prophylaxis for *Pneumocystis jiroveci* (formerly *Pneumocystis carinii)* when CD4 threshold is below 200.
- Start prophylaxis for *Toxoplasma gondii* when CD4 threshold is below 100.
- Start prophylaxis for *Mycobacterium avium complex* when CD4 threshold is below 50.

Treating occupational HIV exposure in healthcare settings

- Percutaneous injury with hollow-bore needle is the most common route of occupational HIV transmission.
- Post-exposure antiretroviral treatment reduces the risk of transmission.
- Healthcare personnel should be offered the maximally potent combination treatment immediately after exposure (preferably within hours, or even minutes).
- Alternately, exposed personnel may prefer to wait until the source patient has documented evidence of HIV infection (using a rapid HIV test).

Acute HIV infection

- Acute HIV infection cannot be determined with standard serologic tests.
- Serologic tests do not become positive until 3–4 weeks after acute infection.
- Diagnosis requires a high index of suspicion.
- Clinical: may see fever, fatigue, rash, headache, lymphadenopathy, pharyngitis, myalgia, or arthralgia.
- Routine lab clues: thrombocytopenia, leukopenia, or elevated liver function tests.
- Diagnosis is made by finding elevated serum levels of viral p24 antigen or viral RNA in a patient with a negative test for HIV-1 antibodies.
- Once the diagnosis has been made, the patient should be offered immediate, maximally potent combination antiretroviral therapy. However, the benefit is not clear, and clinical trials are ongoing.

Zidovudine

- Nucleoside (thymidine) analog that blocks reverse transcriptase (nucleoside reverse transcriptase inhibitor [NRTI]).

Lamivudine

- Another nucleoside (thymidine) analog that blocks reverse transcriptase.
- Trimethoprim/sulfamethoxazole increases bioavailability.
- Has activity against HBV and should not be used as only agent with anti-HBV activity in an HIV regimen; beware of HBV flares if drug is discontinued.

Emtricitabine

- Another nucleoside (thymidine) analog that blocks reverse transcriptase.
- Has activity against HBV and should not be used as only agent with anti-HBV activity in an HIV regimen; beware of HBV flares if drug is discontinued.

Abacavir

- Interferes with HIV viral RNA dependent DNA polymerase.
- Ethanol may increase toxicity.
- Fatal hypersensitivity may occur with reintroduction of abacavir therapy.

Nevirapine

- Non-nucleoside reverse transcriptase inhibitor.
- Different mechanism than zidovudine and lamivudine to inhibit reverse transcriptase.
- Decreases concentrations of protease inhibitors.
- May decrease effectiveness of oral contraceptives.
- Monotherapy causes drug-resistant HIV.
- May cause rash or Stevens-Johnson syndrome.
- Risk of hepatotoxicity, including fatal fulminant hepatitis, particularly in women with CD4 counts greater than 250 and men with CD4 counts greater than 400.

Efavirenz

- Another non-nucleoside reverse transcriptase inhibitor.
- Major side effects are dizziness and insomnia; may also cause depression, suicidal behavior, and paranoia.
- Teratogenic; should not be used in women who are pregnant or may become pregnant.

- Induces hepatic enzymes; caution when used with other drugs metabolized through CYP3A4 pathway.

Tenofovir

- Inhibits reverse transcriptase by substrate competition and by DNA chain termination.

Protease inhibitors

- Lopinavir/ritonavir—lopinavir inhibits HIV protease; ritonavir increases bioavailability of lopinavir; may cause pancreatitis.
- Atazanavir—good gastrointestinal tolerance and minimal effects on lipids; now often used as first protease inhibitor.

Enfuvirtide (Fuzeon)

- First of a new class of anti-HIV drugs known as "fusion inhibitors."
- Blocks HIV from entering the human immune cell by inhibiting gp41 protein.
- Side effect: increased risk of bacterial pneumonia.
- Drawbacks: parenteral administration and very high cost.

Trimethoprim/sulfamethoxazole (Bactrim)

- Drug of choice for *Pneumocystis jiroveci* (formerly *Pneumocystis carinii)* pneumonia.
- Always start prednisone first for PaO_2 less than 70 mm Hg.
- May increase levels of zidovudine.
- Raises INR of patients on warfarin.
- Alternative: Pentamidine for *Pneumocystis jiroveci* pneumonia patients who are allergic to Bactrim.

Amphotericin B

- Drug of choice for cryptococcal meningitis.
- Fever and chills common with infusion.
- May cause hypotension, bronchospasm, arrhythmia, and shock.
- Monitor renal function, CBC, and liver function.

Ganciclovir

* Active against cytomegalovirus (CMV).
* May cause granulocytopenia, anemia, and thrombocytopenia.

Pyrimethamine

* Highly active against *T. gondii*.
* May precipitate hemolytic anemia in glucose-6-phosphate dehydrogenase deficiency.

CHAPTER 22

Poisonings and Overdoses

Gastric lavage

- Consider if patient reaches emergency department (ED) early (within one hour of overdose).
- Contraindicated in acid/alkali burn or hydrocarbon ingestion, or if patient has bleeding disorder.
- Complications include aspiration pneumonitis and esophageal perforation.

Methanol poisoning

- Found in antifreeze and solvents.
- Latent period of up to 24 hours.
- Causes gastrointestinal (GI) and central nervous system (CNS) symptoms including dizziness, headache, and seizures.
- Also causes blurred vision and blindness.
- Lab shows osmolal gap.
- Remember thiamine and folate.
- Treat with IV ethanol or 4-methylpyrazole (blocks alcohol).
- Supplement folinic acid (leucovorin) to help formic acid elimination.
- Hemodialysis for severe cases.

Ethylene glycol poisoning

- Found in antifreeze and de-icing solution.
- Causes GI and CNS symptoms.
- Lab may show osmolal gap.

- Late effects (12–72 hours): pulmonary edema, cardiomegaly, and renal failure.
- Urine may show oxalate crystals 4–6 hours after ingestion.
- Treatment similar to methanol poisoning.

Organophosphate and carbamate poisoning

- Organophosphate and carbamate cause most pesticide poisonings.
- Irreversibly bind and deactivate acetylcholinesterase.
- Causes accumulation of acetylcholine at the neural synapse.
- Headache, muscle cramps, weakness, nausea, vomiting, diarrhea, and excessive secretions.
- Late manifestations are seizure, coma, paralysis, respiratory failure, and death.
- Mainly a clinical diagnosis.
- Treat with atropine (undertreatment is a cause of treatment failure and morbidity).
- Pralidoxime (2-PAM) reverses the phosphorylation of cholinesterase; use to treat muscular weakness.

Carbon monoxide poisoning

- Common cause of poisoning death.
- Clinical presentation may be vague; requires high index of suspicion.
- Diagnose with elevated carboxyhemoglobin level.
- Consider hyperbaric oxygen for severe cases.

Cyanide poisoning

- Results from residential or commercial fire smoke inhalation; industrial exposure such as electroplating; and suicide attempts.
- Sodium nitroprusside in high doses or used for several days can produce toxic blood levels of cyanide.
- Physical signs of cyanide poisoning may be nonspecific.
- Antidotes: nitrites, thiosulfate, and hydroxocobalamin.

Acetominophen (APAP) overdose

- The maximum daily dose is 4 grams in adults.
- Toxic single dose is approximately 7 grams.
- Excess causes hepatocellular death.
- Measure APAP level after *any* overdose (e.g., Darvocet).

- Antidote = *N*-acetylcysteine (NAC); best to administer within eight hours, but never too late (has late protective effects); both IV and PO administration available.

Salicylate overdose

- Can cause a mixed "gap" metabolic acidosis with compensatory respiratory alkalosis.
- Dome nomogram is of limited use and is used less often.
- Can try one activated charcoal dose within first hour.
- Urinary alkalinization is a mainstay of treatment for symptomatic patients.
- Monitor serial arterial blood gasses, urine pH, and electrolytes (including magnesium).
- Hemodialysis is recommended for severe cases (e.g., for altered mental status, renal failure, or pulmonary edema).

Sympathomimetic overdose

- Includes amphetamines, cocaine, aminophylline, pseudoephedrine (over the counter), Ephedra, and 3,4-methylenedioxy methamphetamine (MDMA or "ecstasy").
- Clinical: tachycardia, hypertension, mydriasis (pupillary dilatation), hyperthermia, combativeness, seizure, arrhythmia, diaphoresis, and paranoia.
- No need to follow serial levels. No known antidote.
- Can use benzodiazepines for symptoms.
- Be careful about discharging patients from ED too early; newer, designer drugs can have late effects.

Benzodiazepine overdose

- Extreme sedation.
- Use flumazenil for diagnosis and treatment (very short half life).
- Patients will still require intubation if sedation is refractory.
- Avoid flumazenil in cyclic antidepressant overdose and patients on chronic benzodiazepine treatment (may induce seizures).

Opioid overdose

- Can cause respiratory depression, nausea/vomiting, lethargy, and pulmonary edema.

- Miosis is unreliable (may be absent).
- Often a mixed overdose with other agents (e.g., NSAIDs).
- Use naloxone for significant CNS and/or respiratory depression.

Anticholinergic overdose

- "Red as a beet, hot as a hare, dry as a bone, blind as a bat, mad as a hatter."
- Refers to flushing, fever, dry skin and mucous membranes, mydriasis with loss of accommodation, and altered mental status.
- Occurs after overdose of antihistamines or tricyclic antidepressants.
- Also jimson weed, toxic mushrooms, and certain Chinese herbal teas.
- Antidote is physostigmine; reserve only for severe symptoms (e.g., intractable seizures, severe agitation, etc.).

Lithium overdose

- Clinical: altered mental status, lethargy, seizure, and coma.
- Monitor serum levels at least every two hours.
- Life threatening levels are greater than 2.5 mmol/L for chronic ingestion, or greater than 4.0 mmol/L for acute ingestion.
- Treat with hemodialysis.

Cyclic antidepressant overdose

- Clinical: depressed level of consciousness, hypotension, seizure, and arrhythmias.
- Look for widening of QRS complex on ECG.
- Treat with sodium bicarbonate for evidence of cardiac toxicity.

Selective serotonin reuptake inhibitor (SSRI) overdose

- Clinical: altered mental status, agitation, autonomic dysfunction, tremor, and seizure.
- Prolonged QT interval on ECG most common with citalopram.
- Bicarbonate may help with arrhythmias.
- Seizures most common with citalopram and venlafaxine.

Beta blocker overdose

- Use glucagon to improve positive inotropy.
- Transthoracic or transvenous pacing.
- Consider atropine, epinephrine, or dopamine.
- Insulin and glucose drips to maintain euglycemia.

Calcium channel blocker overdose

- Use 10% calcium chloride single dose (or continuous infusion if refractory).
- Transthoracic or transvenous pacing.
- Consider glucagon with insulin and glucose drip.

Congratulations, you are done with the review book!

- Make sure to go over this book at least two times before the exam.
- Please contact the author with any questions or suggestions for improvement at www.owntheboards.com.
- You are going to do great on your exam!

CHAPTER 23

Practice Mini-Test III

Here is one last quiz to test your knowledge. Make sure to time this test, and please don't look at the answers in the Appendix until you have first completed all of the problems by yourself.

Practice Test III

20 Questions
Time limit: 20 minutes

1. An 18-year-old high-school athlete presents to your office stating that her urine has been blood red for the past 24 hours. Her last menstrual period was two weeks ago. She avoids running when it is hot outside, and drinks adequate water to stay hydrated, but for the last day she felt fatigued, nauseous, and anorexic. History is otherwise negative except for a sore throat two weeks ago. Exam is negative except for a BP of 170/100 and bilateral, mild, lower extremity edema. Pregnancy test is negative. Serum labs show a creatinine of 1.9 g/dL. Urinalysis shows red blood cells, red cell casts, leukocyte casts, and protein. The best diagnostic test is:
   a. Spot urine myoglobin
   b. Serum creatinine kinase
   c. Serum IgA level
   d. Serum anti-streptolysin O

2. A 30-year-old female patient is referred to your office from her OB-GYN for evaluation of asthma with recurrent pulmonary infiltrates on chest x-ray. The patient denies fever, night sweats, hemoptysis, and weight loss. Hemoglobin and creatinine levels are

normal. Pregnancy test is negative. The diagnostic test you should order is:

a. Serum eosinophil level
b. Serum c-ANCA level
c. Skin prick reaction to *Aspergillus*
d. Rigid bronchoscopy

3. A 45-year-old male patient of yours presents to the office complaining of vomiting, diarrhea, and abdominal pain for 12 hours, with associated fever and chills. His symptoms began after a business dinner last night when he was in New Orleans. Physical exam is significant for an ill-appearing man blood pressure of 80/50, and elevated, red lesions on the trunk and the lower extremities. The most likely cause is:

a. *Mycobacterium marinum*
b. *Vibrio vulnificus*
c. Scromboid fish poisoning
d. Tyramine reaction

4. A 55-year-old male salesman presents to your office as a new patient for a complete physical. On history, he states that he suffers from insomnia. He also goes on to relate that his wife nags at him too much and that he was unhappy with the result of the last political elections. Upon further questioning, he states that he is really most bothered by pain in both knees, especially when he has been on his feet all day. On review of systems, he denies suicidal ideation, but states that he has had some sharp chest pains for the last week or two. He goes on to say, "But my wife is the real pain!" Physical exam is unremarkable except for mild hypertension and bilateral crepitus of the knees. The patient appears comfortable and is settling in to his chair so that he can talk with you at greater length. The most important test to order next is:

a. Mini mental status exam
b. Urine toxicology screen
c. Cardiac stress test
d. Knee aspiration

5. A 48-year-old female patient is referred to you with a history of fatigue and pruritus for one month. She also complains of xerophthalmia (dry eyes) and xerostomia (dry mouth). She denies any rash or joint pain. Recent cardiac work up was negative. Past history includes hypertension; the patient takes Captopril. Physical exam is remarkable for mild hepatosplenomegaly. Lab is remarkable for an elevated serum alkaline phosphatase of 450. Abdominal ultrasound

shows a slightly enlarged liver and spleen with normal-appearing intrahepatic ducts. The next best diagnostic test is:

a. Liver biopsy
b. Serum anti-mitochondrial antibody
c. MRI of the liver
d. Serum erythrocyte sedimentation rate

6. A 12-year-old male presents with a three-day history of crampy abdominal pain and bloody diarrhea, which began shortly after eating hamburgers at a summer picnic. Lab is significant for anemia, mild thrombocytopenia, and elevated BUN and creatinine. The most likely cause is:

a. *E. coli* 0157:H7
b. *C. jejuni*
c. *Y. pestis*
d. Shigella

7. A 20-year-old male presents with a solid testicular mass, confirmed by ultrasound. Lab result shows a negative alpha-fetoprotein and negative beta-HCG. Your recommended next step is:

a. Percutaneous biopsy
b. Orchiectomy
c. Staging CT of the abdomen
d. CT chest to rule out pulmonary metastasis

8. A 24-year-old female requests a second opinion from you regarding her recurrent infections with *H. influenza*. The best screening lab test to evaluate her immune status is:

a. CH50
b. C3
c. C4
d. C1 esterase inhibitor

9. A 34-year-old female presents to your office for evaluation of hypertension. On exam, her blood pressure is higher in her right arm than in her left. She also has bounding distal pulses. The most likely diagnosis is:

a. Coarctation of the aorta
b. Takayasu arteritis
c. Renal artery stenosis
d. Primary hyperaldosteronism

10. A 23-year-old, compliant female patient of yours presents for her annual Pap test. She is a non-smoker, and she has taken daily oral contraceptive medication for the past five years. A few days later,

you receive the results of the Pap test, which shows ASCUS. Your next step is:

a. Repeat Pap test in 3–6 months
b. Repeat Pap test in one year
c. Refer for colposcopy
d. Refer for cone biopsy

11. An otherwise healthy 38-year-old gravida 3, para 3, patient of yours presents with a six week history of unilateral nipple discharge from the left breast. Her only medication is ibuprofen for occasional headaches. The nipple discharge is sticky, with multiple colors, but she has never seen bloody discharge. Bilateral breast exam and mammography are normal. Occult blood test on the nipple discharge is negative. Laboratory tests, including a prolactin level, are normal. The most likely diagnosis is:

a. Mammary duct ectasia
b. Fibroadenoma of the breast
c. Pituitary adenoma
d. Breast cancer

12. A 50-year-old, mentally retarded woman is brought to your office by her mother. She takes no medications. The patient has always had poorly developed communication skills. However, the patient has lately been having "bad dreams" and is behaving aggressively toward family members. The next best step is:

a. Reassurance that this behavior is normal in the mentally challenged
b. Begin a mild antidepressant
c. Evaluate the patient for signs of abuse or neglect
d. Begin a mild sedative

13. A 76-year-old male with a history of prostate cancer presents to the emergency department with one week of increasing cough, dark phlegm, and shortness of breath, with intermittent fever. Exam shows tachypnea and decreased breath sounds on the left base. Lab is significant for an elevated WBC and a left lower lobe infiltrate on chest x-ray. Before initiating therapy, which of the following is the most important part of the history to ascertain?

a. Stage of the prostate cancer
b. Family history
c. Smoking history
d. Recent hospitalization

14. You admit a 66-year-old female to the hospital with a one-day history of atrial fibrillation. The patient is otherwise stable. Complete

work-up is significant only for hyperthyroidism. Your next best step is to treat the patient with:

a. A beta blocker and heparin
b. Warfarin
c. Immediate cardioversion
d. Thyroidectomy

15. A 48-year-old man presents to the ED with a two-hour history of substernal chest pain. ECG on admission showed ST elevation in leads V4–V6, with ST depression and inverted T waves in leads II, III, and aVF. The next morning, his ECG shows Q waves, and lab is significant for elevated troponin levels. Two days later, he complains of sharp chest pain that increases when he is in the supine position. Blood pressure is 120/80, pulse is 78, oxygen saturation is 95%, and temperature is 38.3°C (101.0°F). ECG now shows ST elevations in leads V1–V6 and II, III, and aVF, along with diffuse PR interval depression. The cause of his most recent ECG findings are most likely due to:

a. Ventricular septal rupture
b. Cardiac tamponade
c. Acute pericarditis
d. Recurrent myocardial infarction

16. While on call in the ED you see a 26-year-old gravida 1, para 0, at 38 weeks gestation. She states that for the past week she has had severe headaches and epigastric pain. She has had no problems to date, and her last prenatal visit was normal. On exam, she has pitting edema in her lower extremities. Blood pressure is 150/100 mm Hg. Urinalysis shows 2+ protein. Your next step is to recommend:

a. CT of the head with contrast
b. 24-hour outpatient urine collection for total protein and creatinine
c. Strict bed rest at home, blood pressure control with oral labetalol, and re-evaluate in 2–3 days
d. Admit to the OB service for treatment with intravenous magnesium sulfate, blood pressure control, and immediate delivery of the fetus

17. A 52-year-old African American man presents with symptoms of heartburn and dyspepsia for the last three years. The symptoms have gradually become worse over the last year. Antacids and lifestyle changes do not help. Omeprazole 20 mg/day worked initially, but is no longer helping much. He has no family history of cancer. Exam is unremarkable, and lab for *H. pylori* is negative. He has no other medical problems. The next best step is:

   a. Increase omeprazole to 20 mg BID
   b. Begin a trial of ranitidine, 300 mg BID
   c. Order ambulatory pH monitoring
   d. Refer to a gastroenterologist

18. An 82-year-old male patient of yours was admitted to the hospital one week ago for massive stroke. The patient's neurological status has not improved in the past week. He does not respond to stimuli, and he does not have any spontaneous respirations. A consult from a neurologist states that the patient is unlikely to regain consciousness. The patient has a living will with him that was executed in another state. The patient's wife now requests that you withdraw his hydration and nutritional support as outlined in the patient's living will. However, the patient has three adult children present at the hospital. All three of his children are against the idea of withdrawing support of any kind. The most appropriate course of action is:
   a. Withdraw hydration and nutritional support
   b. Honor the unanimous request of the patient's adult children
   c. Consult the hospital ethics committee
   d. Order more tests to give the family time to work out their differences

19. A 28-year-old white female who has been in excellent health comes to you for her annual Pap test. Speculum examination is normal except for a 1.0 cm raised, friable lesion adjacent to the cervix. All previous Pap tests have been normal. The next best step is:
   a. Reassurance
   b. Repeat Pap test in 3–6 months
   c. Refer for colposcopically guided biopsy
   d. Cone biopsy of the cervix

20. You are evaluating a 76-year-old female patient who has symptoms of moderate to severe depression. She states that she is interested in trying an antidepressant medicine for a few months to see if it helps. She does not want anything that will make her too hyper or too sedated. The best medicine to prescribe for this elderly patient is:
   a. Sertraline
   b. Trazodone
   c. Fluoxetine
   d. Imipramine

STOP TEST

Homework Solutions

Q1: *Acid-base #1 solution*
- 7.4 is neutral, but clinical presentation means we need to check for a mixed disorder.
- Primary change is probably *metabolic* (vomiting and uremia are influencing the bicarb in different directions).
- AG = 144 − (99 + 24) = 21. (So you have a "gap" *metabolic acidosis*.)
- DAG = 21 − 12 = 9.
- DAG + bicarb = 9 + 24 = 33. (This is >26, so *metabolic alkalosis* is also present.)

Q2: *Acid-base #2 solution*
- 7.2 is *acidosis*.
- Primary change is *respiratory*.
- AG= 144 − (99 + 22) = 23. (So you have a "gap" *metabolic acidosis*.)
- DAG = 23 − 12 = 11.
- DAG + bicarb = 11+ 22 = 33. (This is >26, so *metabolic alkalosis* is also present.)

Q3: *Acid-base #3 solution*
- 7.18 is *acidosis*.
- Primary change is *metabolic*.
- AG= 142 − (108 + 10) = 24. (So you have a "gap" *metabolic acidosis*.)
- DAG = 24 − 12 = 12.
- DAG + bicarb = 12 + 10 = 22 (no other acid-base disturbance).

Q4: *Acid-base #4 solution*
- 7.55 is *alkalosis*.

- Primary change is *respiratory.*
- AG = 143 − (102 + 16) = 25. (So you have a "gap" *metabolic acidosis.*)
- DAG = 25 − 12 = 13.
- DAG + bicarb = 13 + 16 = 29. (This is >26, so *metabolic alkalosis* is also present.)

Q5: Acid-base #5 solution
- 7.49 is *alkalosis.*
- Primary change is *respiratory.*
- AG = 143 − (107 + 16) = 20. (So you have a "gap" *metabolic acidosis.*)
- DAG = 20 − 12 = 8.
- DAG + bicarb = 8 + 16 = 24 (no other acid-base disturbance).

Q6: Acid-base #6 solution
- A dobutamine echo has an assumed sensitivity of 90% and specificity of 90% for detecting significant coronary artery disease.
- You are considering using the test to screen military pilots. The prevalence of CAD in this population is 5%.
- What % of patients testing positive will actually have the disease?
- What % of patients with normal results will *not* have CAD?

Construct 2 × 2 table

Table 1	First draw the blank 2 × 2 table from memory.	
	CAD Present	CAD Absent
Stress Test Positive	**True Positive** **A**	**B** **False Positive**
Stress Test Negative	**C** **False Negative**	**D** **True Negative**
	Total # with CAD	Total # without CAD

Working backwards from 5%

Table 2	Working backwards from 5%. Note: Your numbers will likely differ.	
	CAD Present	CAD Absent
Stress Test Positive	**True Positive** A	**False Positive** B
Stress Test Negative	C **False Negative**	D **True Negative**
	100	1900

Filling in the blanks

Table 3	Working backwards to fill in the blanks.	
	CAD Present	CAD Absent
Stress Test Positive	**90** A	**190** B
Stress Test Negative	C **10**	**D** **1710**
	100	1900

Positive/Negative Predictive Value
Thus, the PPV $= A/(A + B)$
$\qquad = 90/(90 + 190)$
$\qquad = 32\%$
Then, the NPV $= D/(D + C)$
$\qquad = 1710/(1710 + 10)$
$\qquad = 99\%$

Practice Mini-Test I Answers

1. The correct answer is B. Toxoplasmosis and histoplasmosis are less likely to present with the given CT findings. *Nocardia asteroides*, in contrast, tends to show confluent pulmonary infiltrates. It also aggressively disseminates and can cause brain abscesses. It is relatively common in renal transplant patients. The rapid onset of symptoms and CT findings make malignancy unlikely.

2. The correct answer is C. Serum tryptase level may be elevated for 90 minutes after acute anaphylaxis, but would not be helpful when symptoms occur for 2–3 days. Immunoglobulin (IgG) level may be decreased in common variable immunodeficiency, which would not explain these symptoms. Serum total IgE and eosinophil levels may be elevated in allergic bronchopulmonary aspergillosis, for example, but this patient did not have any characteristic signs or symptoms such as asthma. In this patient, the history of recurrent angioedema after dental procedures, intestinal obstruction, and laryngeal edema (raspy voice) all point to hereditary angioneurotic edema (HANE). This disease is related to a complement disorder, rather than to a mast cell disorder, so C1 esterase inhibitor levels and C4 levels are decreased.

3. The correct answer is C. This patient has no symptoms of asthma, thus easily eliminating that choice. Hypertrophic cardiomyopathy (HCM) is also inherited in an autosomal dominant disorder. It can also cause collapse and sudden death in young people, particularly after vigorous sports. However, exam findings might be remarkable for an apical fourth heart sound and/or a sustained apical impulse, and the EKG often shows ST-T wave abnormalities and/or LV

hypertrophy. Wolff-Parkinson-White syndrome would show a shortened PR interval, a widened QRS complex, and a delta wave. In contrast, this patient had a rhythm strip showing long QT syndrome. The autosomal dominant variant is known as Romano-Ward syndrome.

4. The correct answer is A. This patient has a pH of 7.50, with the major shift apparent in the pCO_2, which by definition means there is a *respiratory alkalosis*. The anion gap is $149 - (84 + 24) = 41$, which defines a gap *metabolic acidosis*. The delta gap = measured anion gap − normal anion gap (12). Thus, the delta gap $= 41 - 12 = 29$. Adding bicarb $= 53$. Since this is greater than 26, it means there is also a *metabolic alkalosis* present (triple acid-base disorder).

5. The correct answer is B. This patient's symptoms may be caused by surreptitious insulin use. Serum IGF-I is a good screening test for a growth-hormone producing tumor. Cosyntropin stimulation tests for adrenocortical axis deficiency. Oral glucose tolerance is used to evaluate hyperglycemia. In contrast, the serum C-peptide can be used to screen for exogenous sources of insulin—the C-peptide level will be undetectable in surreptitious insulin use.

6. The correct answer is D. Polycystic ovarian syndrome includes symptoms of hirsutism and erratic menses from anovulation. Clinical evidence of prolactinoma might include irregular menses and galactorrhea; it can cause signs of hypogonadism in men, but usually not in women. Addison disease is an autoimmune destruction of adrenals, which can give symptoms and signs of bronze skin, nausea, vomiting, and weakness. The patient in question has symptoms of hypogonadotropism and anosmia, also known as Kallmann syndrome.

7. The correct answer is D. This is a case of familial adenomatous polyposis, which invariably leads to colon cancer. The presence of dysplasia on biopsy means that prompt total colectomy is the treatment of choice. Related family members should also be counseled and screened.

8. The correct answer is D. In this case the number needed to treat only requires the pre- and post-treatment success rates. The rest of the data in the question can be ignored. The formula for NNT = 1/(pre − post). Thus, NNT = 1/(.15 − .10) = 1/0.05 = 20.

9. The correct answer is D. Reed-Sternberg (owl's eye) cells have large, prominent nucleoli and are characteristic of Hodgkin disease. Lymphadenopathy on both sides of the diaphragm is classified as

stage III. The lack of constitutional symptoms makes this an 'A' rather than a 'B' stage. The treatment of Hodgkin stage IIIA and above is usually chemotherapy with ABVD.

10. The correct answer is C. Thrombotic thrombocytopenic purpura (TTP) is characterized by the pentad of anemia, fever, thrombocytopenia, renal failure, and neurologic signs. The treatment of choice is plasmapheresis with fresh frozen plasma replacement.

11. The correct answer is C. The dexamethasone suppression test can help in screening for Cushing, but not for Addison disease, which might be suggested by the patient's bronze skin. Anti-Smith antibody is associated with SLE and lupus nephritis, but would not explain this patient's symptoms. This patient has features of hemochromatosis. Ferritin levels can be useful for monitoring ongoing phlebotomy therapy, but the best initial screening test for the disease is transferrin saturation.

12. The correct answer is B. The patient is asymptomatic and has no evidence of active TB. Thus, obtaining cultures and beginning aggressive therapy are not indicated. However, the documented PPD conversion does require prophylactic therapy. The treatment of choice for prophylaxis includes daily isoniazid for nine months.

13. The correct answer is D. Prolonged treatment with ethambutol can cause optic neuritis. Bilateral blurred vision and color blindness are common symptoms. The condition is often reversible with discontinuation of the drug.

14. The correct answer is A. The small amount of urine protein and absence of fatty casts and oval fat bodies make nephrotic syndrome less likely. Acute glomerulonephritis should have shown red blood cell casts in the urine. Diagnosis of prerenal azotemia is supported by fractional excretion of sodium (FeNa) <1.0 %, which this patient does not have. Livedo reticularis and urine eosinophils are seen with atheroemboli, which can be an unfortunate side effect of AAA repair.

15. The correct answer is D. Tricyclic antidepressants, NSAIDs, and muscle relaxers can provide relief for patients with TMJ syndrome. However, this patient has symptoms more consistent with trigeminal neuralgia; the treatment of choice is carbamazepine.

16. The correct answer is C. Stage III colon cancer is treated with 5-FU + Leucovorin. However, this patient had localized stage III rectal cancer, which should be treated with 5-FU + radiation alone. A mass found within 15 cm of the anus is considered to be rectal cancer.

17. The correct answer is B. Alpha-1 antitrypsin deficiency can explain young-onset symptoms of COPD, but will not explain this patient's presentation. Based on the clinical history, you should suspect cystic fibrosis in this patient. An open lung biopsy might well show bronchiectasis, but this is a nonspecific finding, and at any rate there are easier ways to diagnose it (e.g., bronchoscopy or high-resolution CT). Genetic screening for the abnormal cystic fibrosis gene is not part of the diagnostic criteria, but an increased sweat chloride level is.

18. The correct answer is D. This patient suffers from partial absence seizures, which are best treated with ethosuximide.

19. The correct answer is C. Imaging studies of the pituitary or adrenal glands have a low sensitivity for evaluation of Cushing syndrome. A random serum cortisol also has a low sensitivity. The low-dose, two-day dexamethasone suppression test is more specific than an overnight single-dose test and is used to "rule in" or confirm the diagnosis. Twenty-four-hour urinary free cortisol is another option for confirmation. However, when initially screening for Cushing syndrome, the single-dose, overnight dexamethasone suppression test should be performed first (high sensitivity with moderate specificity).

20. The correct answer is D. Valsalva decreases ventricular filling and decreases cardiac output. So Valsalva decreases most murmurs, except HCM and MVP. In addition, this patient has many of the typical presenting symptoms of HCM, including angina, dyspnea, and palpitations.

APPENDIX C

Practice Mini-Test II Answers

1. The correct answer is A. Oral steroids are the treatment of choice for allergic bronchopulmonary aspergillosis. Inhaled steroids are not effective.
2. The correct answer is B (a beta blocker).
3. The correct answer is D. The cause of "geographic tongue" is unknown, and there is no specific treatment. The diagnosis is made by characteristic clinical signs; biopsy is not needed.
4. The correct answer is C. The patient in question has pernicious anemia (Vitamin B_{12} deficiency).
5. The answer is D. Azithromycin is a preferred treatment for community acquired pneumonia, particularly against *Mycoplasma pneumoniae*.
6. The answer is D. This patient has signs of CMV retinitis.
7. The answer is B. Herpes simplex virus is the cause of herpetic whitlow.
8. The answer is B. INH is the recommended prophylaxis for exposure in higher-risk patients.
9. The answer is C. Rimantadine is recommended for prophylaxis in nursing home patients exposed to a flu outbreak.
10. The correct answer is A. Choice A is an "absolute" criterion for diagnosis. Choice B is a "major" criterion for diagnosis. Choice C is a "minor" criterion for diagnosis. Choice D is nonspecific. (Know all the criteria!)
11. The answer is B. Imipenem IV is notorious for causing seizures.
12. The answer is D. Parvovirus B19 is the most likely infectious cause of this transient arthritis.

13. The answer is A. Treatment with both metronidazole and iodoquinol (a luminal agent) is recommended for outpatient treatment of amebic colitis.

14. The answer is A. Repeat treatment with metronidazole is recommended for the first relapse.

15. The answer is A. When the duration of atrial fibrillation is not known, first perform Transesophageal Echocardiography (TEE). TEE will screen for a thrombus; if negative, fine to proceed with cardioversion.

16. The answer is C. Augmentin monotherapy is a preferred medication for infection prophylaxis after a dog bite. Fluoroquinolones should be avoided in children.

17. The answer is C. In most areas, ceftriaxone and vancomycin are the recommended initial, empiric therapy for bacterial meningitis in this age group.

18. The answer is C. Ceftriaxone and gentamicin are both needed for this acutely ill patient with pyelonephritis and hypotension.

19. The answer is C. Pregnancy can cause a false positive screening test in primary syphilis.

20. The answer is B. Metronidazole is the preferred treatment for trichomoniasis.

Practice Mini-Test III Answers

1. The correct answer is D. Serum IgA levels are often elevated in IgA nephropathy, but are not specific or sensitive, and are not useful clinically. The patient's careful attention to hydration, and her nephritic urine sediment, make rhabdomyolysis unlikely, thus eliminating myoglobinuria and elevated serum CK as useful diagnostic tests in this case. This patient presents with an acute glomerulonephritis, most likely triggered by a Group A strep pharyngitis two weeks previously. The serum ASO titer is sensitive and specific in this case.

2. The correct answer is C. Rigid bronchoscopy is rarely used, except in cases of massive pulmonary hemorrhage or for extraction of a foreign body. Serum c-ANCA level is useful in evaluating Wegener granulomatosis, but this patient does not have symptoms or signs of this disease. In this patient we would suspect allergic bronchopulmonary aspergillosis. Elevated serum eosinophils is not diagnostic, but skin prick reaction to *Aspergillus* is.

3. The correct answer is B. *Vibrio vulnificus* is associated with raw oysters, which are popular at New Orleans' restaurants. Disseminated *Vibrio vulnificus* infection has a high mortality and may cause shock, hemorrhagic bullous lesions, and gastrointestinal symptoms.

4. The correct answer is C. This patient's presentation is familiar to many primary care physicians. The challenge is to sort through the rambling history to find the salient points. The patient mentions chest pain in passing, but quickly tries to minimize it. However,

according to the principle of utility, the patient's chest pain (possible unstable angina) requires attention first.

5. The correct answer is B. This patient has a clinical presentation consistent with primary biliary cirrhosis. Anti-mitochondrial antibody (AMA) has a specificity of 98% for this disease.

6. The answer is A. Hemolytic uremic syndrome is most often associated with *E. coli* 0157:H7.

7. The answer is B. Percutaneous biopsy has no role in the diagnosis of testicular tumors; it can alter lymphatic drainage and can "seed" or spill tumor cells. Staging CT is typically performed after diagnosis is confirmed by orchiectomy and pathology. Chest x-ray is probably adequate for screening the lungs for metastases and has a lower false positive rate.

8. The answer is A. CH50 is the best initial test to evaluate classical or terminal complement pathway deficiencies, which can predispose to recurrent bacterial infections.

9. The answer is B. Coarctation of the aorta is characterized by diminished distal pulses and blood pressure differential in arms. However, Takayasu disease has the same symptoms, but can often give bounding distal pulses as well.

10. The answer is A. ASCUS stands for atypical squamous cells of undetermined significance. The question does not give you any information on the patient's human papilloma virus status. The recommendation for ASCUS in a compliant, pre-menopausal patient is to repeat a Pap test in 3–6 months. Less than three months would not provide enough time to develop detectable neoplastic changes and could lead to false negatives. Waiting more than a year to repeat the Pap test is not recommended in ASCUS. If the follow-up Pap still shows ASCUS, at that point you would refer the patient for colposcopy with biopsy.

11. The answer is A. Mammary duct ectasia is a benign lesion of the breast. The mammary ducts become dilated, with associated fibrosis, inflammation, and discharge. Ultrasound often will show ectasia of the ducts.

12. The answer is C. A careful history and physical exam can help to uncover signs of abuse or neglect. That is the first step; a sedative or antidepressant can be offered later if warranted.

13. The answer is D. It is important to determine whether the patient was recently discharged from the hospital, which would change the antibiotic regimen from community-acquired to hospital-acquired pneumonia coverage.

14. The answer is A. The immediate treatment involves anticoagulation with heparin, along with a beta blocker to quickly ameliorate the effects of elevated thyroid hormone. The patient is stable, and thus medical management should be started first, before surgery or cardioversion.

15. The answer is C. The new ECG findings are classic for acute pericarditis.

16. The answer is D. This patient has signs and symptoms of preeclampsia, possibly severe. A CT of the head might show mild edema, but would not change the management. Outpatient workup and treatment is too risky. The preferred treatment for severe preeclampsia is magnesium sulfate to prevent seizure, blood pressure control, and immediate delivery of the term fetus.

17. The answer is D. This patient has symptoms of reflux that are worsening and refractory to proton pump inhibitor therapy. The next best step is referral to a gastroenterologist for EGD, in order to rule out Barrett esophagus, malignancy, etc.

18. The answer is A. The living will speaks for the patient when he cannot, and it takes precedence over the wishes of other family members. The patient's wishes, as expressed in the living will, should be honored.

19. The answer is C. Abnormal lesions visible on speculum exam require a biopsy. However, cone biopsy is more invasive and is not the first step. Instead, colposcopy can give a better view of the lesion, and will allow for a more accurate, and less invasive, initial biopsy.

20. The answer is A. In this elderly patient, trazodone would be too sedating at doses required for treating depression. Imipramine is the least preferred; as a tricyclic, it has the most anticholinergic side effects. Fluoxetine can initially induce anxiety in some elderly patients. Sertraline is therefore the best initial choice and should be tolerated the best in this patient.

INDEX

Page numbers followed by a Q denote questions; those followed by an "A" denote Answers